The Health Care Workforce in Europe

Learning from experience

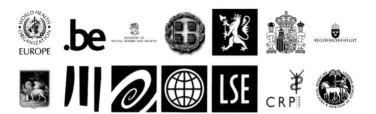

The European Observatory on Health Systems and Policies supports and promotes evidence-based health policy-making through comprehensive and rigorous analysis of health care systems in Europe. It brings together a wide range of policy-makers, academics and practitioners to analyse trends in health care reform, drawing on experience from across Europe to illuminate policy issues.

The European Observatory on Health Systems and Policies is a partnership between the World Health Organization Regional Office for Europe, the Governments of Belgium, Finland, Greece, Norway, Spain and Sweden, the Veneto Region of Italy, the European Investment Bank, the Open Society Institute, the World Bank, CRP-Santé Luxembourg, the London School of Economics and Political Science and the London School of Hygiene & Tropical Medicine.

The Health Care Workforce in Europe

Learning from experience

Edited by

Bernd Rechel
Research Fellow, London School of Hygiene & Tropical Medicine, United Kingdom

Carl-Ardy Dubois
Assistant Professor, Department of Nursing Sciences, University of Montreal, Canada

Martin McKee
Professor of European Public Health, London School of Hygiene & Tropical Medicine, and Research Director, European Observatory on Health Systems and Policies, London, United Kingdom

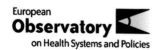

European
Observatory
on Health Systems and Policies

Keywords:
HEALTH OCCUPATIONS – trends
HEALTH MANPOWER – trends
DELIVERY OF HEALTH CARE
COMPARATIVE STUDY
FRANCE
GERMANY
LITHUANIA
MALTA
NORWAY
POLAND
RUSSIAN FEDERATION
SPAIN
UNITED KINGDOM
EUROPE

ISBN 92-890-2297-3

Printed and bound in the United Kingdom by The Cromwell Press, Trowbridge, Wilts.

Contents

Tables, figures and boxes

Tables

Figures

Boxes

About the authors

Natasha Azzopardi Muscat is Director, EU and International Affairs, Ministry of Health, Malta, and Coordinator, Health Services Management Division, Institute of Health Care, University of Malta, G'Mangia, Malta.

Are-Harald Brenne is a Master's student at the Department of Economics, University of Bergen, Norway.

James Buchan is Professor in the Faculty of Social Sciences and Health Care, Queen Margaret University College, Edinburgh, United Kingdom.

Reinhard Busse is Professor and Head of the Department of Health Care Management at the Technical University of Berlin, and Associate Research Director of the European Observatory on Health Systems and Policies, Berlin, Germany.

Kirill Danishevski is Research Fellow at the London School of Hygiene & Tropical Medicine, and Coordinator of Health System Development Research Programmes in the Russian Federation. He is also Assistant Lecturer in the School of Public Health and Health Management (postgraduate), Department of Public Health and Public Health Consultant, Open Health Institute, Moscow, Russian Federation.

Carmen Delia Dávila Quintana is Professor in the Department of Quantitative Methods for Economics and Management, University of Las Palmas de GC, Spain.

Carl-Ardy Dubois is Assistant Professor in the Faculty of Nursing Sciences, University of Montreal, Canada.

Beatriz González López-Valcárcel is Professor in the Department of Quantitative Methods for Economics and Management, University of Las Palmas de GC, Spain.

Kenneth Grech is Assistant Lecturer in Health Services Management, and Honorary Clinical Lecturer in Public Health in the Faculty of Medicine and Surgery, University of Malta, Malta.

Zeneta Logminiene is Deputy in the Department of Expertise and Audit at the Vilnius Territorial Sickness Fund, Lithuania.

Martin McKee is Professor of European Public Health at the London School of Hygiene & Tropical Medicine, and Research Director of the European Observatory on Health Systems and Policies, United Kingdom.

Alan Maynard is Professor of Health Economics in the Department of Health Sciences, University of York, United Kingdom.

Žilvinas Padaiga is Vice Rector for Studies and Professor of Preventive Medicine in the Faculty of Public Health, Department of Preventive Medicine, University of Medicine in Kaunas, Lithuania.

Jack Reamy is Associate Professor at the Department of Health Services Administration at Xavier University, United States.

Bernd Rechel is Research Fellow at the London School of Hygiene & Tropical Medicine, United Kingdom.

Elena Rodríguez Socorro is Lecturer in the Department of Quantitative Methods for Economics and Management, University of Las Palmas de GC, Spain

Liudvika Starkienė is Adviser to the Minister in the Lithuanian Ministry of Health, Vilnius, Lithuania.

Monika Strózik is Administration Supervisor for KPMG, Poland.

Suzanne Wait is an independent health policy consultant, and Director of SHW Health Ltd. She is also Honorary Senior Research Fellow at UCL and Director of Research at the International Longevity Centre-UK, London, United Kingdom.

Susanne Weinbrenner is Senior Research Fellow at the Department of Health Care Management, Institute for Public Health, Faculty of Economics and Management, Technical University of Berlin, Germany.

Foreword

Health care is changing. Ageing populations, new therapeutic possibilities and rising expectations have made the provision of health care much more complex than in the past. Many countries are responding to this challenge, introducing new ways of delivering health care. At the heart of these changes are the health professionals. They must acquire a range of new skills. Some are technical, such as how to get the most from new information systems or advances in technology. Some are organizational, such as how to work in multi-disciplinary teams. Yet the new landscape requires more than this. It also demands new attitudes, finding ways in which the health professional can engage in effective partnerships with both their patients and the organizations that purchase care on their behalf and who look beyond the individual patients to understand the needs of the population.

These changes are taking place at a time of considerable environmental turbulence. This is exemplified by patterns of professional migration. Long-established movements, such as those between the Indian sub-continent and the United Kingdom, are slowing down in the face of new immigration rules. At the same time, there is increasing movement from the countries of central and eastern Europe that joined the European Union in 2004. Within countries, work forces are changing. Traditional gender divisions are breaking down and in many countries women now constitute a majority of new medical graduates. Physicians, who have in the past worked long and often anti-social hours, are demanding a changed work–leisure balance. At the same time, they are having to balance the need to provide round-the-clock cover with the provisions of the European Working Time Directive.

A companion volume by the European Observatory, *Human resources for health in Europe*, looked in detail at the key issues affecting the health workforce in Europe. It drew on a series of detailed case studies undertaken to assess the situation in a range of European countries. This volume brings those case studies together.

The European Investment Bank is proud to be a partner in the Observatory. It is a major investor in the health sector and is committed to ensuring that the projects it supports contribute to an improvement in the health of Europe's citizens. The projects that it supports, such as hospitals and other health facilities, provide the setting in which many health professionals deliver care. The task before us is to integrate the design of facilities with the therapeutic pathways along which patients and health professionals travel.

The case studies contained in this volume provide a means of exchanging information on the challenges that countries face and the solutions that they are exploring. We hope that this sharing of knowledge will be useful to health policy-makers as they work to ensure that the delivery of health care meets the needs of the citizens of tomorrow.

Stephen Wright
European Investment Bank

Acknowledgements

This volume is one of a series of books produced by the European Observatory on Health Systems and Policies. We are grateful to all the authors for their hard work and enthusiasm in this project.

In addition to the work of the authors (see the list of contributors on pages vii–viii), this work draws on *Human resources for health in Europe*, a related volume edited by Carl-Ardy Dubois, Martin McKee and Ellen Nolte. The contributors to that volume, in addition to the editors, were James Buchan, Bonnie Sibbald, Charles Shaw, Anne Mahon, Ruth Young, Alan Maynard, Anne-Marie Rafferty and Anna Dixon (United Kingdom), Suzy Lessof, Carl Afford, Rita Baeten, Yves Jorens (Belgium), Sigrún Gunnarsdóttir (Iceland), Elizabeth K. Kachur (United States) and Karl Krajic (Austria).

We appreciate the contributions of those who participated in a workshop held in Berlin to discuss a draft of the volume. These were, in addition to the case study writers and the chapter authors: Walter Baer, Philip Berman, Auron Cara, Paul de Raeve, Tatul Hakobyan, Gulin Gedik, Galina Perfilieva, Pille Saar, Peter Scherer, Markus Schneider, Noah Simmons, Marjukka Vallimies Patomaki and Lud F. J. van der Velden. We are also grateful to Reinhard Busse and his assistant Patricia Meirelles for hosting and organizing the workshop.

We are especially grateful to the Canadian Health Services Research Foundation for their award of a post-doctoral fellowship to Dr Dubois, and to Jonathan Lomas, its Chief Executive Officer, for his support and encouragement.

We very much appreciated the time taken by the final reviewers, Nigel Edwards and Philip Berman, and we benefited from their helpful comments and suggestions.

Finally, this book would not have appeared without the hard work throughout the project of the production team led by Giovanna Ceroni, with the able assistance of Sue Gammerman, Caroline White and Nicole Satterley.

Bernd Reckel
Carl-Ardy Dubois
Martin McKee

Chapter 1

Introduction: Critical challenges facing the health care workforce in Europe

Carl-Ardy Dubois, Martin McKee, Bernd Rechel

Contemporary health systems are faced with an important paradox. On the one hand, consistent increases in health care investments over past decades and major developments in biomedical research have resulted in an extraordinary expansion of knowledge, technologies, techniques, skills and resources that make it possible to tackle many major health problems more effectively than ever before. On the other hand, many recent attempts to reform the health care sector have had only limited success in the quest to develop a more effective, efficient, safe and equitable delivery system that achieves the fundamental goal of improving population health. One of the major, but often overlooked, factors in the success or the failure of such efforts is the configuration of the health care workforce. The inability to reap the full benefits from current investments in health care results, in many instances, from the difficulties of creating and maintaining an effective, efficient and motivated workforce. A host of problems, ranging from looming shortages of some types of health care workers, accelerating labour migration, and distributional imbalances of various types (geographic, gender, occupational, institutional) to qualitative imbalances (underqualification or misqualification of health care workers) have undermined the capacity of health systems to respond effectively to the challenges they face. This has given rise to a belated recognition of the centrality of human resources for health as the backbone of all health actions (Chen et al. 2004).

As one part of a major study undertaken by the European Observatory on Health Systems and Policies, this book investigates the critical gaps in the health care workforce and their management in nine European countries. It seeks to communicate a sense of urgency to address the many key workforce issues that seriously impede the ability of health systems in Europe to enhance their performance and to achieve their goal of improving population health. To achieve this, it examines the policies that have already been put in place and highlights key areas where appropriate interventions are still needed to ensure an effective development of human resources for health, and the harmonization of policies and practices relating to the health workforce with national health goals.

The comparative study of human resources

Interest in the comparative study of health systems has gained momentum in the past decade as most industrialized countries have been grappling with common concerns. The potential benefits of studying human resource policies and practices from a comparative perspective have been recognized by both academics and practitioners (Clark et al. 2000). Recognition of these benefits has now extended to international comparative research on the management of human resources for health (Dubois and McKee 2006). Comparative studies of human resources provide policy-makers with a valuable knowledge basis for workforce reforms by offering lessons from experiences elsewhere. In the current context of the internationalization of the health labour market, cross-national comparisons have been used by policy-makers to gain a more accurate understanding of where their health care systems rank as employers of choice. Comparative studies also offer a tool to gain new insights into issues facing the health care workforce, whether by expanding observations beyond the parochial limits of national experiences or by demonstrating what is unique about any configuration of national human resource arrangements.

Comparative studies entail a systematic cross-examination of phenomena; they have both descriptive and analytical aspects. The approach taken in this study has been to examine the configuration of the health care workforce and human resource management practices by carrying out case studies of nine European countries. In another book (Dubois et al. 2005), data collected for this study, including the nine case studies, have been used analytically, providing cross-national evidence that can help to identify and explain plausible patterns of similarities and differences in the configuration of the health care workforce. However, we recognize that many policy-makers are interested in the question of what a particular country does, and why some things happen in the same way in some countries but in different ways in others. The present book therefore provides descriptive accounts of the different national experiences that have been used in the comparative study. The nine case studies in this book provide a picture of the health care workforce in Europe and highlight how different countries have dealt with the health workforce challenges they are facing.

Valuing the diversity of Europe

Recent debates about the evolution of the welfare state have been polarized between arguments supporting the convergence of social policies and counter-arguments claiming that divergent national backgrounds contextualize social policies (Dosi and Nelson 1994; Hofstede 1980; Kenneth 2001; O'Reilly 1996). These dichotomous positions have been replicated in the fields of human resource management and health sector reforms (Brewster 1999a; Brewster 2004; Brewster 1999b; Field 1989; Globerman et al. 2001; Gooderham and Brewster 2003).

The convergence argument stresses the importance of a series of factors that are driving public policy reforms and management of the workforce in industrialized countries in the same direction. The power of markets, the pressures for enhanced productivity and quality, the resource constraints faced by all welfare states, the rapid diffusion of similar technologies, and a wide-spread emphasis on benchmarking practices are all seen as contributing to shaping similar policies in different countries, leading towards the adoption of an ideal set of human resource practices that supposedly work in all countries. From this perspective, the increasing economic and political integration of European Union (EU) countries, which has been termed as a process of Europeanization, has been seen as a possible motor of convergence towards a distinct set of European human resource management practices (Brewster 1995).

From the opposite perspective, proponents of the divergence thesis argue that human resource systems reflect national institutional contexts and cultures and do not respond readily to the imperatives of technology or the market. It is assumed that differences in politics, education, labour market and trade unionism are reflected in human resource policies and practices. From such a perspective, the objective is not to look for an ideal set of universal best practices but whether the pattern of human resource activities fits the specific context of the country concerned, and in particular whether it is consistent with that country's policy choices outside the area of human resources.

There is no doubt that Europe provides a specific context within which to explore the field of human resources for health from both of these perspectives. European health systems make up a possibly unique mixture of unifying and dividing elements, with many possible points of comparison at the European level, the level of regional groupings within Europe, and at the regional and local level within each country. The advent of the EU as a project dedicated to large-scale institutional harmonization, the introduction of common regulations and a common currency within a common market are factors that have an impact upon the European health care workforce, its development, its mobility and how it is managed. However, the European perspective is the equivalent of looking through a wide-angle lens. Narrowing the focus to different regions of Europe or different groups of countries offers an opportunity to reveal different models for conducting social policies and managing people. Contributions from different fields (industrial relations, political science and business studies) have turned attention to those regional clusters made up of countries who often share a common legacy associated with history, geography, culture and traditions. Hofstede (1980) distinguished between the Latin, Anglo-Saxon and North European cultures, phenomena reflected in different work-related attitudes. Comparative analyses of labour relations have found distinct models of corporatism and of governance of labour markets prevailing in different parts of Europe: a centralist state tradition in southern Europe (France, Italy and Spain), characterized by state control over key aspects of policy-making and adversarial relations between the state and social partners; a German type of legal corporatism characterized by dispersion of power and influence between statutory public and private organizations; and a Scandinavian institutional tradition characterized by a high level of integration of organized groups within the state and a high degree of cooperation between the social partners (Crouch 1993; Ebbinghaus 1999; Ebbinghaus 2001; Poole 1986; Thelen 2001; Wilsford 1995). Yet, despite similarities between them, countries within a given cluster do not form a totally homogeneous group. In all cases, it is still necessary to further narrow the focus so as to illuminate the political, social, economic, cultural, and legal features that shape policies and practices at both the national and local level within each country.

The countries included in this study provide an appropriate mix to examine the health care workforce in Europe at different levels. Nine countries were selected: France, Germany, Lithuania, Malta, Norway, Poland, the Russian Federation, Spain, and the United Kingdom. Other than Norway and the Russian Federation, all these countries are now members of the European Union. Against the supranational framework of the EU, the historical and social development of these countries is rooted in different institutional traditions. These countries provide a range of approaches to governing the health care workforce. Some of the countries are facing particularly challenging workforce issues requiring policy attention. Others have recently engaged in explicit health care reforms with major implications for their workforce.

The French health system provides a particular workforce management context that mixes liberal elements with a strong government role in assuring universal coverage, regulating the health system and managing a national network of public health care organizations. The enduring ideals of *la médecine libérale*, first formulated in 1928 by a physicians' union, ensure the free choice of physicians by patients, the freedom of physicians to practise wherever they choose, clinical autonomy, doctor–patient confidentiality, and direct payment to physicians by patients (Rodwin and Le Pen 2004). At the same time, the centralization of policy-making means that the Government is given the powerful capacity to control all key aspects of the health care system. The French Ministry of Health is, for instance, the sole decision-maker in relation to the planning policy for the workforce. The professional associations are fragmented and have not developed a strong role as participants in social policy-making. This has led to growing dissatisfaction among health care workers and increasing difficulties in concluding agreements with associations of health professionals (Sandier et al. 2002). For many years the French Government has vigorously applied a system of *numerus clausus* as an effective tool to limit the growth in numbers of health staff. However, the debate has shifted in recent years and there is now a fear of shortages of doctors, nurses and other health care professionals.

Germany is an example of a federal and corporatist system in which health care goals are fixed and implemented within a complex set of institutional mechanisms acting at different levels. Providers and purchasers of health services work within a corporate framework that includes more than 300 sickness funds, 23 regional physicians' associations, 22 regional dentists' associations and their corresponding federal associations (Busse and Reisberg 2000). The corporatist nature of the system is reflected in the many rigidities that make it difficult to introduce changes (Altenstetter and Busse 2005). In this highly fragmented environment, the state, whether at federal or *Länder* level, has traditionally only been able to use a few levers to regulate the diverse aspects of the workforce. As an example, the Government was not able to approach workforce planning by controlling the number of students in medical schools, leading to an overproduction of physicians (Mable and Marriott 2001). However, recent reforms have largely sought to introduce more state intervention, imposing new constraints on corporatist actors. Typical examples include the implementation of global budgets for physician payments, limits on the number of physicians allowed to treat patients insured through sickness funds, and, although ultimately unsuccessful, greater control of budgets for pharmaceuticals.

Lithuania is one of the newly independent states that emerged from the collapse of the Soviet Union. The transition from the Soviet command model of administration to a market-driven economy, accelerated by the EU accession process, involved attempts to replace the former tax-based system of health care financing with a mandatory health insurance model. At the onset of transition, the composition of health care workers and facilities reflected clearly the legacy from the communist era. Human resources for health were characterized by centralized planning, high numbers of staff, a workforce dominated by specialists, the low status of generalists, and the absence of a private sector. A key element of many of the reforms has been the replacement of the old model based on narrow specialties with one of integrated primary care centred on general practitioners, and considerable efforts have been devoted to the training or retraining of general practitioners. The requirements to meet the criteria for EU membership have also driven substantial reforms in graduate education, and postgraduate training and nursing studies have been introduced at university level. However, a persisting oversupply of physicians and prospects of shortages of nurses have recently drawn attention to the urgency of creating a cohesive framework for the development of the health care workforce. As one of the countries with the lowest national income per capita in the enlarged European Union, Lithuania faces a particular threat of losing health professionals through migration to other Member States (Krosnar 2004).

Malta is one of those Mediterranean countries that have historically been characterized by a lower level of economic development than most western European countries. It has a long-standing tradition of openness to influences from abroad, in particular from its former colonial power, the United Kingdom. The accession of Malta to the EU has meant that it has had to address a number of workforce challenges, such as compliance with the Working Time Directive, retention of health care professionals in the face of greater opportunities to work abroad, and updating of professional legislation. The case of Malta also serves to illustrate the challenge of workforce management in a health care system that has traditionally been highly centralized, with nearly all decisions being taken at the level of the Ministry of Health. Within the highly centralized and regulated health system, the process of staff recruitment is centrally controlled and rigid working conditions prevail. The main thrust of health policy in recent years has been directed towards decentralizing power. Yet the management system is still somewhat bureaucratic owing to complex civil service procedures that have an impact on human resource management (Azzopardi Muscat and Dixon 1999). The Maltese health care system consists of a public health care system that covers the entire population. However, the numbers of health professionals available to work within the public health care service and the means of organizing them have always been limiting factors in the enhancement of service provision. Malta's health care system faces a number of specific issues associated with duplication of public and private care, lack of continuity between the various provider settings, relatively poor salaries, excessive working hours, the undersupply of nursing staff, and the shortage of doctors in the junior and middle grades, as most doctors move overseas for higher specialty training. In 2000, a decision was taken to curtail the opening times of certain health centres because of a lack of sufficient numbers of general practitioners working in the public health service (Azzopardi Muscat and Dixon 1999; European Commission 2002a).

With a population of nearly 4.5 million inhabitants, living in a total land area of 386 958 km², Norway is one of the most sparsely populated countries in Europe. This means that many health care staff are clustered in and around larger cities and towns, while there are shortages in more rural, northern areas of the country. The regional distribution of general practitioners and dentists in particular is not satisfactory. Norway also exemplifies a country that has faced difficulties achieving self-sufficiency in health professionals. Although recent government policy has focused on increasing the number of students enrolling at health training facilities, Norway continues to look abroad to recruit health care staff, primarily from other Nordic countries and the three Baltic republics. The Ministry of Health has recently recruited a considerable number of nurses and other personnel from Finland.

Norway shares some important common features with the other Scandinavian welfare states with regard to the development of social policies and management of labour relations. One description of the Scandinavian welfare state model is that it is characterized by a relatively large public sector with many public employees, a high degree of publicly financed welfare provision, a pragmatic and consensus-oriented policy-making process, highly developed corporate representation and negotiation in important policy matters, and a very proactive labour market policy characterized by substantial public spending on employment services, moving allowances, and job training (Blom-Hansen 2000; Erichsen 1995; Esping-Andersen et al. 1992).

Poland is part of the group of post-communist countries in central and eastern Europe that have embarked on democratic transition, economic liberalization and accession to the EU. The process of transition has involved many social and institutional reforms, one of which has been the reform of the health system. A primary intention of the health care reforms was to shift away from the centralized integrated state model (the Soviet-imposed Semashko system) to a decentralized and contracted model of social health insurance, modelled in part on the basic features of the Bismarckian system. To achieve EU membership, Poland also had to adapt its health system in ways that ensured conformity and harmonization with those elements of EU legislation that impinge on health systems. This process of transition has left a very clear imprint on the labour market in Poland. The passage by the Polish Parliament of the Physicians' Chambers Act of May 1989, along with the Pharmacists' Chambers Act and the Nurses' and Midwives' Self-Government Act of 1991, provided the foundations for the development of self-governing bodies and professional organizations of medical personnel (European Commission 2002b). The Nurses' and Midwives' Act and the Medical Profession Act of 1996 determined formal requirements for medical professionals serving within the health care system, but more importantly, they also established the conditions for private practice (European Commission 2002b). As a consequence of developments in health-related legislation, a number of practical changes have also been made in areas such as education and training to ensure equal status for Polish health professionals in the labour market of the enlarged EU (Zajak 2004). Following EU accession, retention of Polish health professionals has emerged as a key policy issue. There are concerns that professional migration to other EU Member States, fostered by the right to free movement within the single market, may result in the loss of some of the youngest and most highly trained health care staff in Poland.

The Russian Federation exemplifies a series of workforce challenges associated with the (re)building of health systems in post-communist states. The Soviet model of health planning and provision that prevailed in the country was characterized by the pursuit of supranational norms, the production of high numbers of human resources, and the maintenance of large numbers of health centres, clinics and hospital beds with relatively high staff-to-bed or staff-to-facility ratios. The triad of lifelong contracts, inadequate accountability and relatively low wages produced a system with few incentives for productivity or efficiency. Recent reforms have attempted to overturn these effects by decentralizing management and financial responsibility and creating incentives for greater efficiency (Danishevski 2005). A number of measures have been initiated to adapt management and training of the workforce to the new challenges facing the Russian health system. Amongst others, the Ministry of Health has supported reforms of the training of general practitioners (Rese et al. 2005), the autonomy of hospital and polyclinic managers, the payment of staff, and systems of planning and regulation. A major difficulty during this transition process is the context of adverse regulatory and working environments, inadequate health care infrastructure, and weak financing mechanisms.

The Spanish case serves to illustrate how weaknesses in workforce policies and management have resulted in serious imbalances between health care workforce supply and demand. The production of excessive numbers of doctors in the past has left a legacy of difficulties, including unemployment among those physicians who have been unable to specialize. Spain has an unemployment rate among doctors of almost 20%. There is also an over-average supply of pharmacists. In contrast, Spain has the fourth lowest ratio in the EU of nurses per 1000 population. In Spain's integrated public health care system the majority of hospitals are publicly owned and most health care workers are salaried public employees. Although formal responsibility for health care is devolved to Spain's 17 regions, regulations governing the payment of health care professionals, labour relations and negotiation of working conditions mirror the civil service system and are established by the central government. This leaves health managers at regional and facility level with limited flexibility in deciding staffing levels, and limited capacity to negotiate incentives and to enforce commitment of professionals to the objectives of a particular institution (Rico and Sabes 1996). While recent reforms have sought to expand the primary care sector, the hospital sector still retains a very high proportion of total health care professionals and there are considerable recruitment and retention issues in the primary care sector and in some geographical areas.

In the United Kingdom, the publicly organized and financed National Health Service (NHS) has initiated two successive reforms with far-reaching implications for human resources for health over the past two decades. From the early 1990s, the Conservative Government under Margaret Thatcher established an internal market with the intention of changing incentives and accountability mechanisms for both purchasers and providers, with the goal of enhancing the system's microeconomic efficiency. The hierarchical managerial relationship between health authorities and providers was replaced with a relationship based on contracting between independent purchasers and providers (Tuohy 1999). In the late 1990s, the election of a Labour government led to a further reorganization of the NHS, with a rhetorical shift from competition and markets to collaboration. The NHS plan in 2000 set out a series of national targets and priorities, linked to an explicit commitment to increase NHS staffing, modernize the regulation of health care professionals and ensure that the health care workforce is appropriately skilled and deployed in sufficient numbers (Department of Health 2000). In the wake of these reforms, the NHS developed a complex system that intended to promote continuing professional development and to implement wide-ranging performance management.

The United Kingdom has also had to respond to a shortage of health professionals. As a consequence, it has been particularly innovative in changing the skill mix of professional boundaries, and recruiting from other countries, so that it provides many examples of both the opportunities and challenges of increasing international mobility.

Examining key issues

The meaning of workforce management is far from clearly established in the literature and there is little agreement regarding the most appropriate categorization of human resource management practices. Some analysts suggest four main issues facing the workforce: acquisition, maintenance, motivation and development (Beer et al. 1985). Others refer to workforce management activities as a sequential process that includes recruitment, selection, performance appraisal, rewards and development (Fombrun et al. 1984). Another approach is a fourfold typology, which brings together four rather different areas: employee influence, human resource flow, reward systems and work systems. One main difficulty facing analysts and policy-makers is the extremely large number of activities involved in workforce management. Consequently, attempting to develop a comprehensive model that accounts for all possible human resource management activities and practices appears a challenging task. One proposition to solve this difficulty has been to map a continuum of workforce management practices that range from being transactional to transformational in nature (Lepak et al. 2005). At one extreme, transactional or operational human resource practices focus on the administrative components of human resource management and comprise most of the day-to-day, traditional, personal management tasks relating, for instance, to recruitment, maintenance of discipline and handling of complaints. At the other extreme, transformational workforce practices refer to strategic and system-wide initiatives that contribute to the accomplishment of the system's objectives and systemic changes. The focus of this study is on transformational practices. In the context of health care, four particular areas have been seen as the linchpin of any effort to overcome contemporary health care crises, reshape the delivery of services, improve equity and access, increase efficiency and raise quality. These areas are: workforce planning and staffing, education and training, performance management, and working conditions (Dussault and Dubois 2003; Martinez and Martineau 1998). In examining these four areas concurrently, the intention is to move away from the traditional fragmented approach to human resource management and to take full account of the synergy of various kinds of human resource interventions to transform the health care system.

Workforce supply

Workforce supply is a pervasive challenge facing policy-makers who must seek both to align the health care workforce with health system goals and to sustain changes that are needed for improving the organization and the delivery of health care. An adequate supply means not only sufficient numbers of all types of health care workers but also an equitably balanced distribution: geographically, by category or type of worker, by specialty, across health care institutions and by gender. As will be illustrated in the case studies, fundamental weaknesses in planning the workforce in the past are manifest through a legion of difficulties: cyclical shortages of many health professionals; widespread vacancies, especially in isolated rural areas; and maldistribution of the workforce, creating difficulties in ensuring an equitable provision of care. These difficulties are more likely to be exacerbated rather than attenuated in the future. Demographic changes in Europe, especially the ongoing process of population ageing, increase demands for health services while simultaneously shrinking the pool of workers available to offer these services. The changing composition of the increasingly female workforce, particularly in medicine, changing lifestyle preferences of health workers reflected in aspirations for a better work–life balance, and the general trend towards early retirement are obvious constraints that will impact on the future supply of health care workers. The ongoing process of integration of EU countries and the removal of many barriers to professional mobility pose a direct challenge to the maintenance of an equitable workforce because of the real potential to deprive some regions and countries of key staff that can be attracted elsewhere by better paid jobs and enhanced working conditions. Given these circumstances, human resource planning in the health sector emerges as a key tool to redress these imbalances. Activity that involves the production, the distribution and the balance of health personnel is not an end in itself. It is rather a process that offers multiple policy levers to develop new modes of health care delivery, to create a health care system that is more equitable and to improve access to essential health care services. For instance, increases in the supply of primary health care professionals, notably family physicians and nurses, are an integral part of efforts in many countries to shift towards a more primary care-led health system.

Beyond the issue of numbers, many activities relevant to the planning of the health care workforce, such as changing the scope of practices, redesigning jobs, and transforming skills and roles of professional groups, are prerequisites to progress on major reforms of health systems. While processes of planning the supply of the health care workforce have traditionally been either absent or narrowly focused, more sophisticated and integrated models of workforce planning that cut across different professional groups and take account of a greater number of factors, such as skill mix, skill substitution, technologies, and working practices, seem to offer a better prospect of contributing to the mission of the health system.

Among the key requirements for human resource planning in the health sector are accurate and comprehensive information systems on the actual number of health care workers and their distribution in the health system. As highlighted in the case studies, in several European countries these information systems are still lacking, so that the picture of the health care workforce remains incomplete and inaccurate. Cross-national comparisons based on World Health Organization (WHO) and Organisation for Economic Co-operation and Development (OECD) databases are complicated by incompatible definitions and the use of full-time equivalent staff numbers in some countries and headcounts or professional registers in others.

Even where comprehensive data on human resources for health are available, there remains the question of how many health care workers are required in a specific national context. A simple comparison with another country provides an inadequate benchmark for establishing whether there is an adequate number of health professionals. In some countries, unemployment among physicians is common, highlighting the importance of national labour markets in regulating the number of health care professionals.

Education and training

The health care workforce's core business is to provide safe, high-quality care that improves the health and well-being of the population that it serves. Thus, human resource management cannot be seen as only a matter of workforce numbers and staff mix. It is also concerned with developing cohesive policies in education and training so as to ensure the health care workforce is knowledgeable, skilled, competent and engaged in lifelong learning. Education and training activities provide opportunities to develop packages of skills that differ from those traditionally offered and a workforce that is oriented towards helping achieve the strategic objectives of the health system. Interdisciplinary education, whereby a group of students from various health-related occupations learn interactively during certain periods of their education has proved to be an effective means of fostering interdisciplinary practice and collaboration in providing health-related services (Greiner and Knebel 2003). Innovative curriculum design offers a powerful tool to reformulate the vision of the health system and better prepare graduates for new and enhanced roles such as promoting a healthy lifestyle for patients, working within interdisciplinary teams, assuming responsibility for a group of persons or a population, and improving the quality of interaction and communication with patients. The provision of care in non-hospital settings, the effective use of clinical information to promote evidence-based practice, the measurement and improvement of quality and satisfaction, and the reporting and reduction of error are all targets valued by current reforms that can be supported by changes in how health care professionals are trained.

Working conditions

Having sufficient numbers of workers optimally distributed who are qualified to perform their job well is only part of the equation and will not automatically result in improved patient care and satisfaction. Of equal importance is the optimal utilization of workers, consistent with their technical and interpersonal skills, and under conditions that promote optimal performance. There is now considerable evidence to support the intuitive view that better working conditions increase the motivation of health workers and create the prerequisites for a more effective workforce. Increased workload, greater stress, and dissatisfaction of health care workers with their working conditions undermine their motivation and health, frequently resulting in poor performance.

Improvements in working conditions of health workers involve a whole range of strategies which potentially affect organizational management structures and processes, communication processes, systems of feedback, an improved allocation of resources, the sharing of responsibilities between different actors, and the overall organization of the service delivery system. Many recent attempts to advance the quality, efficiency and equity of health systems have very evident links to improved working conditions. Typical efforts of this nature include attempts to develop incentive systems that support health goals. Financial and other incentives for health professionals are used to alter patterns of clinical practice and to encourage a distribution and use of resources more in line with public needs and collective objectives. Mechanisms to allocate resources and remunerate providers can be used to foster a better balance between activities focusing on prevention and primary care and those relating to curative care. Many innovative strategies that include supportive working environments, personal development, flexible and family-friendly working practices, job enrichment, appropriate working hours, fringe benefits such as housing and day care, and educational opportunities are seen as ways to transform the overall context in which health workers deliver their services, enhance their motivation and consequently improve the overall performance of the health system.

Performance management

Performance management relates to the optimization of the service production process so as to make sure that staff are encouraged to provide effective, efficient, high-quality services that will meet the needs and expectations of citizens. Managing performance of health care workers involves a whole set of institutional and incentive arrangements that cut across the different functions of the health systems (funding, provision, resource generation, and stewardship) and look to influence their performance (WHO 2000). The setting of practice standards and quality assurance programmes, the division of work, the design of payment methods, and the creation of reporting mechanisms are all tools that contribute to the achievement of the functions of health systems, stimulating or enforcing compliance by individual practitioners with appropriate performance standards. Managing performance is also concerned with maintaining technical proficiency in the face of continuous technical and clinical change, ensuring that work processes are as congenial as possible in the light of the nature of the services provided, and developing monitoring systems that foster accountability of both provider organizations and individual practitioners, while avoiding the creation of perverse incentives and opportunistic behaviour. The increased emphasis on the provision of various forms of information (league tables, consumer reports, scorecards, public performance reports, provider/practice profiles, billing patterns), the development of performance indicators, and the strengthening of licensing and accreditation institutions are typical of efforts that are being deployed to make progress towards the achievement of health objectives through mechanisms of performance management targeted at health care workers.

Regulation

Regulation is a common thread running through many changes that affect the entire health system and its workforce. It appears obvious that the regulatory context is a critical element in understanding new forms of health care organization and in the development of new ways to organize and manage the health care workforce. Prevailing practices in planning for the supply of personnel, educating and training the workforce, managing personnel performance and labour relations often cannot change significantly without modifications in regulations and legislation. Regulation provides a powerful tool to shape the market for health services and the behaviour of health care workers through a range of activities that go beyond the traditional self-regulation model and include establishing numbers of personnel to be trained; defining functions to be performed by each category of personnel; issuing personnel policies, stating the regulatory requirements that must be satisfied to practise a profession; negotiating general conditions of work (salary scales and meritorious increases, promotions and career mobility, continuing education); and creating incentives for practitioners to improve their performance and adopt the most cost-effective and evidence-based practices. Depending on the nature of the prevailing political and economic system and the degree of decentralization, these functions will be centralized or shared to varying degrees with lower administrative tiers and with different stakeholders.

Defining the scope of human resources addressed in this book

In *The world health report 2000*, human resources for health were defined as the stock of all individuals engaged in promoting, protecting or improving the health of populations. Such a definition departs from the traditional focus on those formally employed in health systems, especially frontline service providers who come into direct contact with clients (nurses, doctors, pharmacists and other professionals). It reflects recognition of the contribution of a range of less visible health care workers (such as cooks, accountants and archivists) who make the delivery of services possible by providing support to frontline providers. It also draws attention to the broad range of informal providers such as traditional healers, volunteers, and community workers who also make a significant contribution, particularly to community-based support services. Given this broad scope of human resources in health care and the large number of professions and occupations that make up the formal health care workforce, it would be unrealistic to plan a detailed examination of the overall scope of human resources for health within a single study. Pragmatically, this project has focused primarily on the two main health care professions, physicians and nurses. Physicians play a primary role in delivering a full range of essential health services and their influence on the organization of health care and the use of health care resources places them at the centre of health care delivery. Nursing, as the largest professional group in any health care system, deserves a particular emphasis as it undertakes tasks in all areas of health services and provides a complex mix of roles incorporating functions as diverse as caregiver, educator, coordinator, integrator, manager, counsellor and agent of change. Both medical and nursing work are highly sensitive to health care reforms and changes in the health care environment. However, health professions are also characterized by a strong interdependence among multiple professional groups. As a consequence, the practice of physicians and nurses and the outcomes of their work are influenced by the contributions of many other professions and occupations that fulfil important functions in the delivery of health services. Thus, while focusing on physicians and nurses, this research has also sought to document relevant issues related to other health occupations. Special attention has been paid to health care managers (including physician and nurse managers), who play a critical role in both the smooth running of health services and the implementation of many policies that impact on the health care workforce.

The following chapters will look at the experiences of the nine countries in detail.

REFERENCES

Altenstetter C, Busse R (2005). Health care reform in Germany: patchwork change within established governance structures. *Journal of Public Health Politics, Policy and Law*, 30(1–2): 121–142.

Azzopardi Muscat N, Dixon A (1999). *Health care systems in transition: Malta*. Copenhagen, WHO Regional Office for Europe, on behalf of the European Observatory on Health Care Systems.

Beer M et al. (1985). *Human resources management*. New York, NY, Free Press.

Blom-Hansen J (2000). Still corporatism in Scandinavia? A survey of recent empirical findings. *Scandinavian Political Studies*, 23(2): 157–181.

Brewster C (1995). Towards a European model of human resource management. *Journal of International Business Studies*, 26(1): 1–21.

Brewster C (1999a). Different paradigms in strategic HRM: Questions raised by comparative research. In: Wright P et al., eds. *Research in personnel and HRM*. Greenwich, CT, JAI Press: 213–238.

Brewster C (1999b). Strategic human resource management: The value of different paradigms. *Management International Review*, 39: 45–64.

Brewster C (2004). European perspectives on human resource management. *Human Resource Management Review*, 14: 365–382.

Busse R, Reisberg A (2000). *Health care systems in transition: Germany*. Copenhagen, WHO Regional Office for Europe, on behalf of the European Observatory on Health Care Systems.

Chen L et al. (2004). Human resources for health: overcoming the crisis. *Lancet*, 364: 1984–1990.

Clark T, Grant D, Heijltes M (2000). Researching comparative and international human resource management. *International Studies of Management*, 29(4): 6–23.

Crouch C (1993). *Industrial relations and European state traditions*. Oxford, Clarendon Press.

Danishevski K (2005). Case study: Russia. In: Dubois CA, McKee M, Nolte E, eds. *Human resources for health in Europe*. Buckingham, Open University Press.

Department of Health (2000). *The NHS Plan. A plan for investment, a plan for reform*. Norwich, The Stationery Office.

Dosi G, Nelson R (1994). An introduction to evolutionary theories in economics. *Journal of Evolutionary Economics*, 4(3): 153–172.

Dubois CA, McKee M, Nolte E, eds. (2005). *Human resources for health in Europe*. Buckingham, Open University Press.

Dubois CA, McKee M (2006). Cross-national comparisons of human resources for health – what can we learn? *Health Economics, Policy and Law*, 1: 59–78.

Dussault G, Dubois CA (2003). Human resources for health policies: a critical component in health policies. *Human Resources for Health*, 1: 1.

Ebbinghaus B (1999). Does a European social model exist and can it survive? In: Huemer G, Mesch M, Traxler F, eds. *The role of employer associations and labour unions in the EMU*. Aldershot, Ashgate: 1–26.

Ebbinghaus B (2001). European labour relations and welfare-state regimes: a comparative analysis of their elective affinities. In: Ebbinghaus B, Manow P, eds. *Comparing welfare capitalism: social policy and political economy in Europe, Japan and the USA*. London, Routledge.

Erichsen V (1995). Health care reform in Norway: the end of the profession state? *Journal of Health Politics, Policy and Law*, 20: 719–737.

Esping-Andersen G, Eivind Kolberg J (1992). Welfare states and employment regimes. In: Eivind Kolberg J, ed. *The study of welfare state regimes*. Armonk, NY, ME Sharpe.

European Commission (2002a). *Study on the social protection systems in the 13 applicant countries. Malta. Country report*. Brussels, Employment and Social Affairs, European Commission.

European Commission (2002b). *Study on the social protection systems in the 13 applicant countries. Poland. Country report*. Brussels, Employment and Social Affairs, European Commission.

Field MG (1989). *Success and crisis in national health systems: a comparative approach*. New York, Routledge.

Fombrun CJ, Tichy NM, Devana MA (1984). *Strategic human resource management*. New York, Wiley.

Globerman S, Hodges H, Vining A (2001). Canadian and US health care systems performance and governance: elements of convergence. *Applied Health Economics and Health Policy*, 1(2): 75–88.

Gooderham P, Brewster C (2003). Convergence, stasis or divergence? The case of personnel management in Europe. *Beta*, 17(1): 6–18.

Greiner AC, Knebel E (2003). *Health professions education: a bridge to quality*. Washington, DC, National Academies Press.

Hofstede G (1980). *Culture's consequences*. London, Sage.

Kenneth P (2001). *Comparative social policy*. Buckingham, Open University Press.

Krosnar K (2004). Could joining the EU club spell disaster for the new members? *BMJ*, 328: 310.

Lepak D, Bartol K, Erhardt N (2005). A contingency framework for the delivery of HR practices. *Human Resource Management Review*, 15: 139–159.

Mable AL, Marriott J (2001). *Steady state: finding a sustainable balance point – International review of health workforce planning*. Ottawa, ON, Health Human Resources Strategies Division, Health Canada.

Martinez J, Martineau T (1998). Rethinking human resources: an agenda for the millennium. *Health Policy and Planning*, 13: 345–358.

O'Reilly J (1996). Theoretical considerations in cross-national employment research. *Sociological Research Online*, 1: 1 (http://www.socresonline.org.uk/socresonline/1/1/2.html).

Poole M (1986). *Industrial relations: origins and patterns of national diversity*. London, Routledge and Kegan Paul.

Rese A et al. (2005). Implementing general practice in Russia: getting beyond the first steps. *BMJ*, 331: 204–207.

Rico A, Sabes R (1996). *Health care systems in transition: Spain*. Copenhagen, WHO Regional Office for Europe, on behalf of the European Observatory on Health Care Systems.

Rodwin VG, Le Pen C (2004). Health care reform in France – The birth of state-led managed care. *New England Journal of Medicine*, 351(22): 2259–2262.

Sandier S et al. (2002). France. In: Dixon A, Mossialos E, eds. *Health care systems in eight countries: trends and challenges*. Copenhagen, WHO Regional Office for Europe, on behalf of the European Observatory on Health Care Systems: 31–46.

Thelen K (2001). Varieties of labour politics in the developed democracies. In: Hall PA, Soskice D, eds. *Varieties of capitalism: the institutional foundations of comparative advantage.* Oxford, Oxford University Press: 71–103.

Tuohy CH (1999). *Accidental logics: the dynamics of change in the health care arena in the United States, Britain and Canada.* New York, Oxford University Press.

WHO (2000). *The world health report 2000. Health systems: improving performance.* Geneva, World Health Organization.

Wilsford D (1995). States facing interests: struggles over health care policy in advanced, industrial democracies. *Journal of Health Politics, Policy and Law,* 20(3): 571–613.

Zajak M (2004). Free movement of health professionals: the Polish experience. In: McKee M, MacLehose L, Nolte E, eds. *Health policy and European enlargement.* Buckingham, Open University Press: 109–129.

Chapter 2

France

Suzanne Wait

Setting the context

Funding of the French health care system is based on the principle of health insurance, financed mainly by the social security contributions of residents in employment, supplemented with funds from taxation. There are three main schemes: general, or *Caisse nationale d'assurance maladie des travailleurs salariés*, or CNAMTS, covering 84% of the population; agricultural workers, covering 7.2% of the population; and non-agricultural self-employed workers, covering 5% of the population. There are also a variety of smaller schemes such as for the military, doctors in state service, students and miners (Rodwin 2003). Membership is based on occupation and all residents are enrolled in one of the funds in their district (*département*). Since January 2000, a universal health insurance scheme (*Couverture médicale universelle*) has provided financing for the 1% of the population formerly left out of the social security system. It provides free supplementary cover to people whose monthly income is below US$ 580 (Or 2002).

France spends approximately 10% of its gross domestic product (GDP) on health care and in terms of health expenditure is second in the European Union (EU) only to Germany, in terms of health expenditure (OECD 2005); this level has remained relatively stable over the past five years.

Out-of-pocket payments account for about 11% of total health care. Ambulatory patients have to pay for treatment at point of contact and are then partially reimbursed by their local sickness fund (on average up to 70%). To cover the discrepancy, approximately 90% of residents also have supplementary insurance, provided either by a mutual fund (*mutuelle*) or by private insurance. Hospitals are paid directly by sickness funds, and hospital care is reimbursed at 75% (with a cap) and licensed medicines at 50%. Patients with conditions such as pregnancy, AIDS, cancer, diabetes or other chronic diseases are exempt from any co-payment (*ticket modérateur*) (Or 2002). Attempts by successive governments to increase the patient co-payment in order to reduce demand for ambulatory health care services, and thus lower costs, have been unsuccessful (Lancry and Sandier 1999).

Delivery of health care in France is a public/private mix divided into three sectors: an ambulatory sector, containing predominantly office-based practices; a private sector (*secteur libéral*); and a hospital sector that includes:

1 public hospitals, which make up 65% of all hospital beds, are responsible for research and training and are obliged to provide care to anybody in need;

2 private for-profit hospitals (proprietary), which specialize in medium- to long-term care; and

3 private non-profit hospitals, which specialize in surgical procedures.

(DREES 2001; Rodwin 2003).

France has high levels of health care resources (more than 3.4 practising physicians and 3.8 acute hospital beds per 1000 people) and health care consumption (OECD 2005). High-cost equipment tends to be concentrated in public teaching hospitals, and the national government is responsible for ensuring an equal supply and distribution across the country.

The French health care system is highly centralized, and the Ministry of Health in Paris is responsible for managing the provision, financing and monitoring of the quality and costs of health care, and decision-making generally. The central government regulates the supply of health personnel (through a system of *numerus clausus*) and of equipment and medicines. It also sets national training schemes for professionals and establishes quality regulation across all institutions. Since the 1990s social care and long-term care of elderly and disabled people have been organized mainly at district level (Or 2002).

Improvements in the coding system for medical procedures and prescriptions and the consolidation of all reimbursement claims into an electronic database (*Système information d'assurance maladie*) at the CNAMTS have allowed for unprecedented system-wide evaluations of health care utilization patterns (Wait et al. 2000).

Much of the focus of reforms over the past 20 years has been on cost-containment rather than on the quality of treatment, with few government initiatives. Notable exceptions were of the Juppé plan in 1996 and the *Projet de loi de santé publique* (public health bill) in 2003, tackling the actual organization or management of the health care system (Rodwin 2003). This overall approach has contributed to significant tensions between the many sectors involved in health care (Rodwin 2003; Wilsford 1991).

The French health care system faces a number of significant challenges:

* outcomes of care in terms of morbidity and mortality from several chronic illnesses are good, but public health outcomes remain mediocre compared to other European countries (Assemblée Nationale 2002);

* France has one of the highest rates of alcohol consumption in Europe;

* tobacco use among the young is a growing problem;

* premature mortality rates in men are amongst the highest in Europe, mostly due to a high incidence of road traffic injuries;

* socioeconomic inequalities are particularly alarming. Premature mortality is 2.4 times higher for unskilled workers than professionals (Mesrine 2000).

Social and regional inequities are compounded by disparities in the quality of care across providers and institutions (Hémon and Jougla 2003).

Workforce supply

In 2001 health professions accounted for approximately 1 675 000 jobs in France. A general overview of the distribution of human and health care resources across the health care system is presented in Table 2.1. and Table 2.2.

There has been an overall increase of around 30.6% in health workers in France since 1985. The number of physicians has tripled in 40 years, to 332 per 100 000 at the beginning of 2001, and the supply of physicians grew on average by 3.8% per year in the 1980s, and by 1.6% in the 1990s (Mission démographie des professions de santé 2002).

The *numerus clausus* policy has continually decreased the number of students allowed to undergo medical training since it was introduced in 1971. However, notwithstanding this policy, it is estimated on the basis of current physician retirement patterns that the number of practising physicians will remain stable at around 196 000 for a few more years (Niel 2002). If the *numerus clausus* is fixed at its current rate of 4700 students per year, then the medical workforce will decrease to 158 000 at the beginning of 2020, moving from a density of 335 to 253 doctors per 100 000 population (Mission démographie des professions de santé 2002).

Table 2.1 *Distribution of human resources in the French health care system (1998–2002)*

Resources	Rate/figure (year)
Active physicians per 1000 population	3.3 (1998)
Active physicians in private practice per 1000 population	1.9 (2002)
General/family medicine, %	53.3 (2002)
Obstetricians, paediatricians, internists, %	7.5 (2002)
Other specialists, %	39.2 (2002)
Non-physician personnel per acute hospital bed	1.9 (2001)

Source: Rodwin 2003.

Table 2.2 *Distribution of health care resources in the French health care system (1998–2002)*

Resources	Rate/figure (year)
Total inpatient hospital beds per 1000 population	8.5 (1998)
Short-stay hospital beds per 1000 population	4.0 (2000)
Proportion of public beds, %	64.2 (2000)
Proportion of private beds, %	35.8 (2000)
Private for-profit beds as a percentage of private beds, %	56 (1999)
Non-profit beds as a percentage of private beds, %	44 (1999)
Proportion of private for-profit beds, %	44 (1999)

Source: Rodwin 2003.

Women represent 76% of the overall health professional workforce, and this proportion is growing. 36% of doctors are women, and this rate is expected to reach 42% by 2010 (Niel 2002); 35.8% of GPs and 37% of specialists are female. Women already constitute a majority (56%) amongst physicians under the age of 34 years (Mission démographie des professions de santé 2002). The proportion of women in different medical specialties and care settings is presented in Table 2.3.

A key characteristic of the current health workforce is the ageing process. Workers aged less than 35 years only represented 29% of the workforce in 2001 (compared to 52.5% in 1983), and the proportion of middle-aged workers (35–50 years of age) has risen. The proportion of workers over the age of 55, however, has remained stable. Assuming a constant *numerus clausus*, this proportion will gradually start to increase in 2020 when the large cohorts of doctors graduating between 1974 and 1994 start to retire. The average age of practising physicians was 46 in 2001, 44 for women and 47 for men (Mission démographie des professions de santé 2002).

Table 2.3 *Proportion of women according to medical specialization and setting of care*

	Total	Density per 100 000 population	Women (%)	Private sector	Women (%)	Salaried physicians in hospitals	Women (%)
General practitioners	98 505	165	36.8	67 880	28.0	16 463	47.9
Specialists	102 895	173	37.5	52 204	32.2	41 368	38.3
Medical specialties	56 171	94	38.8	28 750	35.3	25 124	40.6
Surgical specialties	24 025	40	23.0	15 973	24.5	7 648	18.8
All physicians	201 400	338	37.2	120 084	29.8	57 831	41.1

Source: ADELI database, 2003. Adapted from Sicart (2003).

The hospital is the main place of work for health professionals, accounting for 45% of all jobs, with an increasing number of doctors beginning their careers in hospitals (Vilain and Niel 2001). Overall, two-thirds of hospital personnel work in the public sector, 27% in private for-profit hospitals and only 8% in private non-profit hospitals (Brahami et al. 2002). 75% of non-clinical hospital staff, as well as approximately 75% of hospital-based nurses, are employed by public sector hospitals (Brahami et al. 2002).

Amongst physicians, the split between private practice (*secteur libéral*) and salaried positions varies by specialty. Since 1985 approximately 40% of physicians have been working exclusively on a salaried basis. Others are either in private practice or in mixed practice (salaried and private practice). 40% of physicians in ambulatory practice work in group practices (Bouet 2003).

70% of general practitioners work in private practice, whereas the split is more even for specialists. Only 30% of general practitioners are employed on a salary-only basis, and this proportion has been increasing for the last five years (Niel 2002). 72% of salaried physicians work in hospitals (Mission démographie des professions de santé 2002).

Efforts to even out the geographical distribution of physicians have been successful over the past few years. There is still, however, a large difference in the availability of physicians, particularly of specialists, between Paris and the southern regions (highest density) and the north of the country (lowest density).

Migration of health professionals into France from the rest of the EU has not yet become significant and very few French physicians undertake their medical training in another EU country, although a significant number of nurses have trained abroad (Mission démographie des professions de santé 2002). There are two possible schemes for foreign-trained physicians from outside of the EU to practise in France, and the best estimates of the numbers so trained are 7000–8000 (3%). Data from 2000 suggest that 1.7% of new doctors received their medical training from outside the EU (CREDES 2001). Migration to France of health professionals other than nurses or physicians is negligible and very few French-trained physicians seek employment abroad.

France has for several years treated a number of patients from the United Kingdom, Italy and North Africa, while French patients, especially those residing close to the border, are treated in other European countries.

In terms of expected future demographic trends, health professionals can be included in one of the following categories:

• physicians, whose numbers will decrease significantly in the years to come;

• dentists, pharmacists and speech therapists, whose numbers will fall in the short term;

• other health professions, including nurses, midwives and physical therapists, whose numbers should continue to increase over the next 10 years.

(Mission démographie des professions de santé 2002)

Education and training

Medicine, pharmacy, dentistry, midwifery, physical therapy and speech therapy are all subject to *numerus clausus*. To enter medical school, a *baccalauréat* is required. After the first year of medical studies, students are required to take an examination that determines whether they can remain in medicine (Mission démographie des professions de santé 2002).

Basic nurse training, into which entry is competitive after completing secondary school, takes three years, with subsequent, optional specializations in theatre nursing, paediatric nursing and anaesthesia taking 9, 12 and 24 months respectively (Sandier et al. 2004).

Continuing medical education is heterogeneous across France. In 1996 it became mandatory for doctors in private practice. Successive governments have altered the framework of continuing medical education, so that there is no central organization accountable for its delivery or evaluation.

Working conditions

Health professionals in France are increasingly reporting dissatisfaction with their working conditions, complaining of a heavy workload, the low status of health care workers (in particular nurses), the rise of medical consumerism, and administrative and legal constraints on practice. Many also report feelings of insecurity about their future. Factors contributing to this are the ageing of the health profession population, the feminization of the workforce, the increasing burdens of illness posed by an ageing population, and changes in the social security system (Mission démographie des professions de santé 2002).

There has been an overall trend amongst health professionals (with the exception of general practitioners and specialists) away from individual practices to shared ones, allowing for more flexibility in scheduling, shared overhead expense and more security in financial returns.

A key issue facing the French health care system is the private–public interface. Public hospitals are financed by global budgets, and tend to deal with more intensive and chronic care, whereas private sector physicians are remunerated on a fee-for-service basis, and thus assume a major role in high-technology diagnostic and other procedures for which there is high added value per treatment. Continuity of care often suffers as a result, as, for example, a cancer patient may be operated on in the public sector, have his/her chemotherapy in a private sector hospital, but receive radiotherapy in yet another hospital (Mission démographie des professions de santé 2002; Wait et al. 2000).

Strategies to coordinate the relationships between public and private health care have been explored at great length but their implementation has yet to become operational (Mission Démographie des professions de santé 2002). Sharing office space, hospital equipment and facilities between public and private health care is the most common model. Since private beds are not "individualized", a patient can change from one sector to the other without actually changing hospital beds depending on the status of his/her treating physician.

Although private–public partnerships in health care have not been very successful, networks of care, involving different health professionals and usually centred on the treatment of one particular condition (e.g. cancer or diabetes), have been more successful in bringing together the private and public sectors.

Remuneration

Hospitals

Private for-profit hospitals are financed on a fee-for-service basis and are paid on the basis of daily rates and fee-for-service payments for specialists, whereas private non-profit hospitals are mostly financed by prospective global budgets, except for 150 hospitals which are paid on a fee-for-service basis (Brahami et al. 2002). Physicians practising in public hospitals receive a salary, but they are also allowed to undertake private practice outside the hospital (Or 2002).

On average, remuneration levels are higher in the public sector than in the private for-profit sector. Private sector hospitals have repeatedly reported difficulties in recruiting health professionals (Brahami et al. 2002). Across all hospital staff, there is a gap of 7–15% in favour of public sector hospitals (Brahami et al. 2002).

Although public hospital personnel may be better paid than their private hospital counterparts, public hospitals are suffering from severe budget cuts. Moreover, in the Government's proposed new hospital plan (*Le plan hôpital 2007*), activity-based payments, similar to resource-based relative value systems used in the United States, are being proposed for payment.

Private practices

Physicians in ambulatory, private practice (*secteur libéral*) get paid by patients on a fee-for-service basis according to a national fee schedule. Doctors who agree to charge on the basis of the nationally negotiated fee are operating in sector 1 and get their social security contributions, including their pension, paid for by the CNAMTS, whereas those who wish to charge higher fees must join sector 2. These fees are subject to a ceiling and the doctors must purchase their own pension and insurance coverage. Patients pay physicians up-front for services and then submit a claim to their local sickness fund to obtain reimbursement for a given percentage of the physician fee. As sickness funds only reimburse the agreed sector 1 fee, patients who consult sector 2 physicians are responsible for the difference in payment. However, this difference is paid for by supplementary insurance for 85% of the population (Or 2002).

The net average salary for a physician in France is about US$ 55 000, less than one-third of their United States counterparts (US$ 194 000) (Audric 2001; Rodwin 2003).

Working hours

The slight increase in the average working time of physicians, from 48 hours per week in 1990 to 51 hours in 2001 (DREES 2001; INSEE 2001), is beginning to reverse and is expected to decrease by two hours over the next 20 years, partly due to the increasing proportion of women in the medical profession, and the increase in doctors aged 55 or over and their choices about work–leisure balance (Mission démographie des professions de santé 2002).

The enforcement of the 35-hour working week, or *réduction du temps de travail* (RTT), took place in early 2000 in private hospitals and in 2002 in public hospitals, but has remained optional. Hospitals that allow their staff to work 35 hours benefit from a 10% decrease in their mandatory social security contributions for employees, and are allowed to hire an additional 6% of staff, which is hoped to lead to an overall gain in productivity (Ségrestin and Tonneau 2002).

Studies found that generally there was satisfaction with the policy, especially the increased leisure time resulting from the RTT, but that work conditions had often not improved. There was an increase in work intensity, less personal contact time with patients, and less flexibility for work schedules, possibly compromising the delivery and quality of care. In public hospitals, professionals felt that previously short-staffed areas were now suffering unduly and there were growing waiting lists and absenteeism.

Retirement

Until 2001, a regulatory measure called MICA (*Mesure d'incitation à la cessation anticipée d'activité*) allowed for permanent retirement at the age of 57 but this measure has been revoked and the number of permanent retirements from practice has been stable since 2000 (Mission démographie des professions de santé 2002).

Performance management

The concept of regulation and external scrutiny was introduced in earnest in 1996 with the *Plan Juppé*, which also marked the beginning of serious recognition of the importance of health care evaluation in France. Several different initiatives were started in the late 1990s in an effort to boost the health care system's regulation of quality:

- improved information systems to facilitate the collection of data on the quality and costs of care;

- the introduction of systematic accreditation both for hospitals and for ambulatory care, under the auspices of the newly founded agency ANAES (*Agence nationale d'accrêditation et d'évaluation en santé*);

- strengthening of continuing medical training and introduction of "ceilings" or targets to control overall spending;

- the adoption of mandatory clinical practice "references" to shape clinical practice (Or 2002).

The ANAES is the main evaluative body in France. It has a clear mandate to "establish the state of knowledge on diagnostic and therapeutic procedures and to contribute to improving the quality and safety of clinical care" (Or 2002). The areas it covers are health technology assessment and evaluation of new technologies, economic evaluation and evaluation of clinical practice. It set up a system of accreditation for all public and private hospitals in France in 1998, following a 1997 decree on hospital reform (Or 2002).

Sickness funds also have an important role in evaluating the quality of care in hospitals and in ambulatory care, they are represented in the regional hospital boards, or *agences régionales d'hospitalisation* (ARH), and help develop and implement regional health strategic plans (*Schéma régional de santé*). They also play an important role in assessing and promoting efficient and appropriate medical practices amongst practitioners in the ambulatory sector.

The evaluation of performance and quality amongst ambulatory sector physicians became a recognized priority with the publication of a decree of 28 December 1999; responsibility for this falls on regional medical unions, the *unions régionales des médecins libéraux,* or URML (Or 2002). Physicians in private practice volunteer to have the quality of their care evaluated, and these evaluations are organized by the ANAES and URML, using local physicians who have been trained as "accreditors".

Clinical guidelines and practice recommendations are to a large extent developed by the professional medical societies, and more than 20 of these societies have organized over 100 conferences during the past 10 years (Or 2002).

In the hospital sector, some hospitals have developed internal quality assurance tools, following the lead of the *Assistance publique-hôpitaux de Paris.* A clinical guideline programme was developed to evaluate and compare hospitals' clinical practices in diagnosis and treatment (Durieux and Ravaud 1997; Or 2002).

National practice recommendations or *références médicales opposables* (RMOs) were first introduced as a concept in the national medical contract in 1993 (the so-called *Loi Teulade*, 1993). In 1996, RMOs were implemented to identify treatments and prescriptions which were considered to be dangerous or judged ineffective. There are currently 155 RMOs, with which general practitioners must comply. The RMOs need to be evidence-based and formulated in such a way that the criteria for evaluation and sanctions are absolutely clear. Although provisions for sanctions against doctors who failed to comply with RMOs were specified in 1998, these sanctions were abolished in 1999 and 2000 (Or 2002).

Regulation

As mentioned above, *numerus clausus* was established in 1971 as a regulatory system to restrict the number of medical students. There is no system of regular revalidation or recertification.

The reforms introduced in the late 1990s aimed to improve quality and to contain costs. However, these two objectives often became confused in the minds of practising physicians. Some authors even claim that the focus on cost-containment had a direct negative impact on the implementation of guidelines (Or 2002). For example, the *Plan Juppé* stipulated that physicians should be subject to collective sanctions if they overspent the budget approved by parliament. Eventually this policy was considered to be unconstitutional and was revoked but efforts to evaluate and regulate quality and costs lost credibility in the process (Or 2002).

A huge obstacle facing policy-makers wishing to contain costs or enforce system-wide evaluation or regulations in France is the fee-for-service payment system for physicians in private practice. This, combined with the fact that patients have complete freedom of choice of physician, means that doctors perceive themselves to be at financial risk if they refuse to prescribe what a patient requests. Financially, there are absolutely no incentives for physicians to reduce the number of prescriptions they hand out.

The main regulatory body for hospital care is the ARH. The ARH are responsible for the management and strategic planning of both public and private hospitals and also play a role in ensuring the equitable distribution of hospital care within each region. The ARH place a huge emphasis on quality, and this is used as a criterion in negotiating hospital budgets. Hospitals are bound by a contract which sets out specific objectives and targets (*Contrat d'objectifs et de moyens*) and specifies areas where investment is needed to improve the quality of care. Quality is assessed using the ANAES accreditation framework as well as by the *agences régionales d'hospitalisation* based on specific criteria. Since 1999, all public and private hospitals must have a specific committee responsible for observing the quality of hygiene, which must develop a plan for monitoring and reducing hospital infections (Or 2002).

Conclusions

Over the past 30 years the number of health care workers in France has grown continuously but this trend is now due to reverse over the next 30 years. This decrease in the projected health care workforce comes at a time when demographic factors such as ageing will affect both the supply of health professionals and the demand for health care. Moreover, the impact of the EU Working Time Directive and changing working patterns in favour of fewer working hours may contribute to threatening the quality of care and the overall functioning of hospitals throughout the country. The *plan hôpital 2007* which has been proposed by the French Government does not fully resolve how the health system is going to cope with increasing demand and diminishing supply.

The strength of the health care system is its ability to facilitate flexible working patterns for physicians and other professionals, and the scope for collaboration between private and public sectors, hospitals, private clinics and professional practices to pool resources and to work towards the efficient delivery of services. However, intersectoral and hospital–private practice collaborations have not yet found the means to achieve true economies of scale.

The French system combines complete freedom for professionals to choose where and how they practise their profession, with tight regulation and centralization of authority within the Government and sickness funds. This tension has dominated the workings of the health care system for years, and becomes apparent every time national physician contract (*convention*) negotiations take place between medical unions, sickness funds and the Government. Nonetheless, budgetary constraints, the growing recognition of the importance of regulation, and evaluation to ensure the quality of care, may help to lessen these tensions in the years to come.

France has only recently embraced the notion of evaluation in earnest. The recently proposed public health law (*Projet de loi de santé publique*) promises to invest heavily in public health and to significantly build up the epidemiological information base throughout the health care system to allow for continuous monitoring of outcomes. Access to computerized information on utilization practices at the CNAMTS (via the *Système informatique de l'assurance maladie*) has considerably reinforced the capacity for evaluation and quality improvement within the health care system.

A special government committee proposed that an observatory be set up to continuously survey the demographic situation of health professionals. This would provide a continuously updated picture of the demographic situation of health professionals across the country, and would recognize when significant gaps between supply and demand needed to be addressed (Mission démographie des professions de santé 2002).

Methods for projecting the numbers of health professionals have so far remained simplistic, and only the data on physicians have been harmonized successfully from different sources. The impact that extraneous factors may have on the numbers of health professionals in the future must be ascertained. Moreover, consideration of factors affecting individual specialties would be more valuable than the existing overall projections based on the total number of physicians. Similarly, forecasts of the numbers of physicians and health professionals based on national figures provide little help to iron out issues with supply, where discrepancies exist at the district level within the country.

A key question that remains is what criteria to use when deciding what the "optimal" level of supply of professionals should be. One can use historical precedents, international and subnational comparisons, but it is naive to assume that the national average is necessarily the optimum for the entire country. This challenge will become particularly meaningful in the years to come, as professional numbers decrease throughout the French health care system.

REFERENCES

Assemblée Nationale (2002). *Projet de loi politique de santé publique.* Paris, Assemblée Nationale (http://www.assemblee-nationale.fr/12/rapports/r1092.asp).

Audric S (2001). *Les disparités de revenues et de charges des médecins libéraux.* Paris, Direction de la recherche, des études, de l'évaluation et des statistiques (DREES), Ministère de l'Emploi et de la Solidarité (Etudes et Résultats, No. 146).

Bouet P (2003). *Liberté d'installation, liberté d'exercice. Quelle médecine pour quels médecins? Rapport de la Commission nationale permanente adopté lors des Assises du Conseil national de l'Ordre des médecins du 14 juin 2003.* Paris, Ordre des médecins (http://www.conseil-national. medecin.fr/?url=rapport/article.php&offset=2).

Brahami A, Brizard A, Audric S (2002). *Les rémunérations dans les établissements de santé privés.* Paris, Direction de l'animation de la recherche, des études et des statistiques (DARES), Direction de la recherche, des études, de l'évaluation et des statistiques (DREES), Ministère de l'Emploi et de la Solidarité (Série Etudes, Document de travail, No. 25).

CREDES (2001). *Démographie médicale: peut-on évaluer les besoins en médecins?* Paris, CREDES (Rapport No. 1341).

DREES (2001). *Le temps de travail des médecins.* Paris, Direction de la recherche, des études, de l'évaluation et des statistiques (DREES), Ministère de l'Emploi et de la Solidarité (Etudes et Résultats, No. 114).

Durieux P, Ravaud P (1997). From clinical guidelines to quality assurance: the experience of Assistance Publique Hôpitaux de Paris. *International Journal for Quality in Health Care*, 9: 215–219.

Hémon D, Jougla E (2003). *Estimation de la surmortalité et principales caractéristiques épidémiologiques. Surmortalité liée à la canicule d'août 2003 – Rapport d'étape*. Paris, Institut national de la santé et de la recherche médicale (INSERM) (http//:www.sante.gouv.fr/htm/actu/ surmort_canicule/rapport_complet.pdf).

INSEE (2001). *Enquêtes emploi*. PARIS, Institut Nationale de la Statistique et des Etudes Economiques (http://www.insee.fr/fr/home/home_page.asp).

Lancry P, Sandier S (1999). Rationing health care in France. *Health Policy*, 50(1–2): 23–38.

Mesrine A (2000). La surmortalité des chômeurs: un effet catalyseur du chômage? *Economie et Statistique*, 334(4): 33–49.

Mission démographie des professions de santé (2002). (http://www.demo-profsante.pdf).

Niel X (2002). *La démographie médicale à l'horizon 2020. Une réactualisation des projections à partir de 2002*. Paris, Direction de la recherche, des études, de l'évaluation et des statistiques (DREES), Ministère de l'Emploi et de la Solidarité (Etudes et Résultats, No. 161).

OECD (2005). *Health data 2005*. Paris, Organisation for Economic Co-operation and Development (http://www.oecd.org).

Or Z (2002). *Improving the performance of health care systems: from measures to action (a review of experiences in four OECD countries)*. Paris, Organisation for Economic Co-operation and Development (OECD Labour Market and Social Policy Occasional Papers, No. 57; http://ideas.repec.org/p/oec/elsaaa/57-en.html).

Rodwin VG (2003). The health care system under French national health insurance: lessons for health reform in the United States. *American Journal of Public Health*, 93(1): 31–37.

Sandier S, Paris V, Polton D (2004). *Health care systems in transition: France*. Copenhagen, WHO Regional Office for Europe, on behalf of the European Observatory on Health Systems and Policies.

Ségrestin B, Tonneau D (2002). *La réduction du temps de travail dans les établissements privés sanitaires, médico-sociaux et sociaux*. Paris, Direction de la recherche, des études, de l'évaluation et des statistiques (DREES), Ministère de l'Emploi et de la Solidarité (Etudes et Résultats, No. 171).

Sicart D (2003). *Les professions de santé au 1er janvier 2003*. Paris, Direction de la recherche, des études, de l'évaluation et des statistiques (DREES), Ministère de l'Emploi et de la Solidarité (Document de travail, No. 52).

Vilain A, Niel X (2001). *Les médecins hospitaliers depuis le début des années 80: davantage de débuts de carrière à l'hôpital*. Paris, Direction de la recherche, des études, de l'évaluation et des statistiques (DREES), Ministère de l'Emploi et de la Solidarité (Etudes et Résultats, No. 145).

Wait S, Schaffer P, Blanchard O (2000). La prise en charge hospitalière du cancer du sein dans le Bas-Rhin. *Journal d'Economie Médicale*, 18(2): 85–100.

Wilsford D (1991). *Doctors and the state: the politics of health care in France and the United States*. Durham, NC, Duke University Press

Chapter 3
Germany

Susanne Weinbrenner, Reinhard Busse

Context

Although one of the largest economies in Europe, Germany has faced increasing budgetary pressure in recent years, owing to high unemployment, changing demographics and the costs of German reunification. Germany spends a comparatively high share of its national wealth on health, ranking third among OECD countries in 2003, with 11.1% of its GDP spent on health (OECD 2004). With respect to health spending per capita, Germany ranks seventh but the increase in real terms accounted for only 1.3%, far below the OECD average of 4.5%. In December 2003, 4.2 million people were employed in the health care sector, constituting 10.7% of the German workforce, according to data from the Federal Statistical Office (Federal Statistical Office 2003a).

Health care financing is based on a system of statutory health insurance, comprising multiple sickness funds, that covers almost 87% of the population, with a further 10% of the population (those above a certain income can opt out of the otherwise mandatory system) covered by private health insurance (Federal Statistical Office 2003b). A further mandatory insurance programme (*Pflegeversicherung*) was introduced in 1994, in order to ensure access to nursing care for elderly people. All members of statutory sickness funds (including pensioners and unemployed people), as well as people with comprehensive private health insurance, were compulsorily enrolled in the new insurance scheme, making it the first social insurance programme with population-wide membership.

Statutory health insurance is the major source of health financing, accounting for 56.7% of overall health expenditure in 2003. Other mandatory insurance systems, including mandatory care insurance, contributed a further 6.9%, while government sources contributed 7.8%.

The German health system is based on the principles of federalism and corporatism. Most legislation has to be approved by the Federal Council (*Bundesrat*), the legislative assembly of the 16 states (*Länder*) that constitute the Federal Republic of Germany. The states are also responsible for inpatient care, emergency and public health services, medical education and the supervision of professional associations.

Providers and purchasers of health services work within a corporate framework, and include more than 300 sickness funds, 23 regional physicians' associations, 22 regional dentists' associations and their corresponding federal associations. Membership of the respective professional associations is mandatory and each has a democratically elected structure and the right to raise its own financial resources. Regional physicians' and dentists' associations are obliged to ensure the provision of ambulatory care throughout the 24-hour period. They negotiate collective contracts with the numerous sickness funds that operate in their state and distribute the financial resources they receive among their members. A substantial part of decision-making is decentralized. Corporatist decision-making usually takes place in joint committees of sickness funds and provider associations, addressing issues such as benefit coverage, quality assurance, and reimbursement and accreditation of providers.

The sickness funds are the purchasers in the social health insurance system. Since 1996, most insured persons have the right to choose their sickness fund freely. Funds are obliged to enrol any applicant, in order to minimize cream-skimming. In 1995/1996, a risk structure compensation scheme was established, compensating funds for differences in the cost profile of their insured. In addition to recurrent costs, sickness funds also cover the maintenance costs of hospitals, while capital investments in the hospital sector are financed by the states.

Ambulatory care is mainly provided by private providers working in single practices. Patients have free choice of physicians, dentists, pharmacists, emergency care, and, since 1998, psychotherapists. Reimbursement of care by other health professionals, including hospital care, is available following referral by physicians.

The organization of health services in Germany was changed with the Health Care Reform Law of 1989. The law diminished the powers of the regional associations of physicians and sickness funds, resulting in a reduction of their legitimacy and innovative power. Nevertheless, the health system continues to be organized according to the principles of federalism and corporatism on the basis of collective contracts.

Following the reunification of Germany, inequities in health and health care between the two parts of the country have been reduced substantially by large-scale government investment (Advisory Council 2001). One of the remaining concerns in relation to health financing is the increasing gap between income and expenditure of sickness funds. Although there have been attempts to slow down contribution rates for mandatory health insurance since the 1970s, all of these measures have failed to achieve sustainable savings, while overall health expenditures increased. The average contribution rate increased from 12.4% of gross salary in 1991 to 14.2% in 2004. One of the reasons for this increase is demographic change, with an ageing population and a decrease in health insurance revenue.

Workforce supply

Data on the German health care workforce differ significantly according to source. According to OECD data, the health care workforce accounted for 6.8% of total employment in 2001 (OECD 2004). A significantly higher percentage of total employment, 10.3% in 2001, was recorded by the Federal Statistical Office (Federal Statistical Office 2003a). This discrepancy might be due to the fact that the figures were based on different units (head counts versus full-time equivalents). For the year 2003, the data do not differ substantially: 10.6% (OECD 2005) versus 10.7% (Federal Statistical Office 2005).

According to statistics from the Federal Statistical Office, in 2003 42% of health personnel were working in inpatient facilities, 41% in outpatient facilities, 7% in industry and laboratories and 5% in administration. The share of part-time workers has increased in recent years, accounting for about 29% of health personnel in 2003, 91.7% of whom were women (Federal Statistical Office 2005) .

Table 3.1 provides data on the numbers of selected medical professionals per 100 000 population according to the European Health for All database. As shown in Table 3.1, the number of all health professionals increased between 1991 and 2003, with the highest increases among physicians and nurses or midwives (until 1997 nurses and midwives were counted together). The number of dentists and pharmacists increased considerably in the first half of the 1990s, but the increase has since levelled off. For physicians, dentists and pharmacists, the number of graduates shows a downward trend, in particular since the second half of the 1990s.

Table 3.1 *Medical professionals 1991–2003 (per 100 000 population)*

	1991	1993	1995	1997	1999	2001	2003
Physicians	279	292	307	313	321	331	337
Dentists	69	72	74	76	76	78	78
Pharmacists	52	53	55	57	58	58	58
Nurses/Midwives	885	867	900				
Nurses				924	949	973	
Midwives				9.3	9.0	9.5	
Graduate physicians	12	15	15	11	10	8.5	
Graduate dentists	2.5	2.3	2.2	2.3	2.3	2.2	1.7
Graduate pharmacists	2.8	2.9	2.6	2.0	1.8	1.5	

Source: WHO 2005.

Physicians

As is the case with the total number of health professionals, data on the number of physicians vary significantly according to data source. The OECD, for example, excludes physicians outside the inpatient and outpatient sectors from the category of "practising physicians", while the Federal Physicians Chamber and the European Health for All database include them. Even more obscure are (implicit) definitions of general practitioners and specialists. OECD and WHO databases overestimate the number of general practitioners and specialists, as they understate the number of physicians without specialization, many of whom are in training to become a specialist.

According to the Federal Physicians Chamber, the number of practising physicians increased by about 20% during the 1990s, reaching a ratio of 3.63 per 1000 population in 2001. Since then numbers have fallen, with 2.69 practising physicians per 1000 inhabitants in 2004. The density of physicians is much lower in rural areas and in the eastern states. The lowest density of physicians, at 2.84 per 1000 population, was recorded in the state of Brandenburg, while in Hamburg there were 5.32 physicians per 1000 population. In rural areas, there are up to five times more patients per physician than in urban areas. The number of physicians contracted by the health insurance system has been regulated by law, mainly to prevent an oversupply in urban areas. In many rural areas, there is an insufficient number of general practitioners, in spite of efforts to increase supply.

Another problem facing the physician workforce is ageing. The share of physicians younger than 35 years decreased from 27.4% in 1991 to 18.8% in 2000. Between 1993 and 2001, the average age of physicians in ambulatory care increased by about three years. The number of women accepted for registration has increased continuously over the last decades, reaching 45.6% in 1999, although, for reasons that remain unclear, women still constitute only 36.8% of working physicians. The proportion of women is particularly low in some specialties, such as surgery, where only 12.5% of specialists are female. The representation of women is even lower in managerial positions.

Physicians' associations distinguish between 36 main groups of specializations. For these, the Federal Physicians' Chamber has established training programmes, which are further specified by the regional physicians' chambers. Following their initial training, physicians are required to pass an examination in their specialty. To the extent that data are comparable, the supply of specialists in Germany is above the European average. According to the OECD, there were 2.2 specialists per 1000 population in Germany in 2001, a figure that is 10% lower according to the Federal Physicians' Chamber.

In the 1980s, the growth in the number of physicians was considered to be a major cause for spiralling health expenditures. Sickness funds and physicians' associations demanded a reduction in the supply of physicians by reducing the number of medical students and limiting access of physicians to the mandatory health insurance system. The bypassing of general practitioners by those consulting specialists was identified as another upward pressure on costs, as the typical consultation with specialists is much more expensive than a consultation with a general practitioner. The gatekeeper function of general practitioners has subsequently been strengthened, but there is still no comprehensive system of human resource planning.

While the emigration of physicians has not played a significant role in recent years, an increasing number of physicians have migrated to Germany. In 2001, 15 143 physicians from abroad were registered in Germany. 10% came from the former Soviet Union, 10% from Iran, 7% from Greece, 5% from Turkey, 4% from Austria, 4% from the former Yugoslavia and 4% from Poland. Immigration is encouraged by good job prospects. In February 2002, a new record number of unfilled positions was recorded (3800), equivalent to 1.3% of the number of practising physicians.

Nurses

Accurate data on the number of nurses in Germany are lacking, since nursing is not considered to be a profession and nurses do not need to register with a particular organization. However, there has been a trend towards a professional-ization of nursing over the last decade. More than two-thirds of all nursing professionals and those working in related social services have completed three years of formal training. Nursing science has now been established as a university discipline, with 50 different courses of study in Germany. There are

Table 3.2 *Nursing workforce 1997–2002 (full-time equivalent, in thousands)*

	1997	1998	1999	2000	2001	2002	% change 1997–2002
Trained nurses	528	532	528	526	526	539	+2
Nurse assistants	152	150	154	162	165	170	+12
Nurses caring for elderly patients	151	160	174	187	199	211	+40
Total	831	842	856	875	890	920	+11

Source: Federal Statistical Office 2003a.

currently 24 universities of applied sciences offering courses on nursing management or nursing education.

At present, a monitoring system for the assessment of nurses on the basis of professional qualifications and experience is lacking, as is a system of human resource planning that considers future nursing needs. The Health Care Structure Law of 1993 introduced nursing time standards, in order to overcome perceived nursing shortages. A standardized unit of nursing time was allocated to nine categories of patients, allowing calculation of the predicted nursing time for each ward. The nursing time standards resulted in the creation of almost 21 000 new nursing positions between 1993 and 1995. As this increase exceeded the expectations of policy-makers, who had anticipated an increase of only 13 000 nursing positions during this period, nursing time standards were discontinued following a new law in 1997. Nevertheless, the overall number of full-time equivalent nurses increased by a further 11% between 1997 and 2002. This increase was, however, to a large extent due to the introduction of the mandatory care insurance scheme in 1994, which led to an increase of 40% in the number of nurses caring for elderly people (see Table 3.2).

Unfortunately, there are no data available on the geographical distribution of nurses or on specialization within the nursing profession. According to national nursing associations, only 10% of nurses are organized in professional associations. Of all nurses, about 15% are male and 42.6% are less than 35 years old. The majority of nurses (about 82% of full-time equivalents in 2002) are working in hospitals, but the number of nurses in nursing homes and in institutions providing ambulatory nursing care has grown more rapidly in recent years.

As is the case with physicians, there tends to be a higher ratio of nurses to patients in bigger hospitals. The best-staffed hospitals are general hospitals with more than 500 beds, with an average of 33.7 physicians and 81.5 nurses per 100 occupied beds. In general for hospitals with fewer than 100 beds the corresponding average figures are 13.7 physicians and 66.4 nurses (Arnold et al. 2003).

So far without success, the umbrella organization of nursing associations in Germany has been demanding corporatist status for the nursing professions. If this status were achieved, nurses could play a role of equal importance to physicians' associations in the governance of the health system.

Health managers

Health managers are still a young profession in Germany and they are not accounted for in official personnel statistics. The situation is, however, changing. Until recently, the management of hospitals was supervised by executive committees consisting of representatives of physicians, nurses and administrators, with the medical director having the most influence. Nowadays, hospitals are generally managed by a managing director.

Other health professions

Since 1999, psychologists working in the ambulatory care sector as "psychological psychotherapists" have been recognized as a new occupation, with the same status in the mandatory health insurance system as physicians. Psychologists working as psychological psychotherapists have been organized in professional chambers since 2003.

Apart from the regular health care professions whose services are paid by public funds, Germany has a unique state-regulated profession – the *Heilpraktiker*, or "alternative practitioner", offering complementary and alternative medicine. Health professionals who want to practise as *Heilpraktiker* need to obtain a state licence, as set out in federal law. In contrast to other health professions in Germany, the law specifies what these health professionals are *not* allowed to do, aiming at preventing fraud and harm to the health of the population. Most *Heilpraktiker* are self-employed and have their own practices, although more detailed data on this profession are lacking.

Main challenges of supply

Until 2002, the supply of medical services in hospitals was largely unregulated. The heads of departments decided on the therapies to be offered, while there was no specified catalogue of services. Since 2003, the reimbursement of hospitals has been changed to one based on diagnosis-related groups (DRGs). Through this change, hospitals have been forced to reorganize their services and the management of their workforce. The change in the reimbursement of hospitals is expected to strengthen the trend among physicians and nurses to pursue higher qualifications.

A shortage of staff to provide care for elderly people outside hospitals has been one of the main political topics relating to human resources in the health sector in recent years. Policy-makers reacted to demands from consumer organizations and carers by adopting the Law on Quality Assurance and Consumer Protection in Care in 2001.

As already mentioned, there is also an inadequate supply of ambulatory services by physicians in some areas of the country. Physicians' associations have been expected to improve the performance of their members, but regulatory instruments aimed at improving the quality and provision of physicians' services remain weak.

Education and training

In line with the federal political structure of the country, the states are generally responsible for regulating and financing education, and for registering and supervising professions. Traditionally, health professions differ from other professions in two aspects: undergraduate medical education is regulated at federal level, and medical chambers possess virtual autonomy in regulating specialist and continuing education.

Many German universities offer degrees in medicine, dentistry and/or pharmacy. Over the last five to seven years, the number of first-year medical students has remained constant at around 9700. The total number of students, however, has decreased by 11.3%, while the number of graduates has decreased by about 23%, as approximately 20% of those enrolled each year do not finish their medical studies (Kassenärztliche Bundesvereinigung 2001; Kassenärztliche Bundesvereinigung 2002).

Most university places are distributed centrally according to school marks, a medical entry test, waiting times and special quota (such as for people from abroad and people with disabilities). The remaining 15% of places are allocated by universities following individual interviews.

University studies last between four years for pharmacy and six years for medicine. The curriculum is highly standardized and organized around three to four central examinations. However, since 1999 medical faculties have been allowed to offer revised curricula. The first reformed curriculum started in 1999 at Berlin Humboldt University. In autumn 2002, a new regulation for the licensing of physicians was issued by the Federal Ministry of Health and approved by the Federal Council. The regulation aims to facilitate bedside teaching and has an orientation towards primary care, problem-solving skills and the integration of science with clinical subjects. After graduation, medical doctors were required to work 18 months in clinical practice before being eligible for full registration. Owing to an increasing shortage of physicians, this regulation has effectively been abolished since 1 October 2004. All other health professionals can obtain registration at the relevant state ministry responsible for health immediately after their graduation (Kälble 2002).

In 1999, there were about 1050 centres for nurse training, offering about 69 000 training places (Arnold et al. 2002). In the same year, there were 4467 training places for physiotherapists and 787 places for speech therapy (Arnold et al. 2002).

For 16 out of 22 non-academic health care professions, uniform curricular frameworks have been established. Undergraduate training of most non-academic health professions requires an advanced school degree after secondary school and usually takes three years. It is generally organized within the framework of vocational education, with on-the-job training and teaching in vocational schools.

The main problems facing the educational system for nurses and related social services are their position in the vocational educational system, the lack of flexibility of the educational infrastructure, outdated course content, a shortage of qualified teaching personnel and the distinction between the educational systems for nurses and social service personnel. Nurses, paediatric nurses and nurses caring for elderly people continue to be trained separately.

Education of both academic and non-academic health professionals is free of charge, when provided in state institutions. Participants in vocational education, such as nurses, receive a basic income during training. University education is financed by the states, while practice-based training at hospitals is generally funded by statutory insurance funds within the framework of their contracts with individual hospitals.

While medical graduates are in reality obliged to specialize, at least if they want to work independently, specialization is optional for other health professionals. Practice-based specialization usually takes two to three years in non-academic and four to six years in academic health care professions. The duration of specialization in general medicine was increased from three to five years in 1998, in order to strengthen the status of general practitioners. In addition, trainees in general medicine have received incentives during their training period. Licensing as a psychological psychotherapist requires three years' full-time or five years' part-time training in state-approved institutions. Public health used to be exclusively a medical specialty, but has now been introduced at nine universities as a postgraduate course. Quality management is another part-time qualification which has been introduced in recent years. Continuing professional education is voluntary, with self-regulation by professional associations (Kälble 2003).

Several universities have introduced courses on economics for physicians. The University of Hanover has established a master's degree in health care management and there are several universities offering master's degrees in business administration. Eight universities have set up courses leading to a master's degree in public health, three universities are offering a joint course leading to a master's degree in epidemiology and the University of Heidelberg is offering a course in community health and health management in developing countries.

Dropout rates from professional training and practice are particularly high for non-academic health professionals. Possible reasons include a failure to take account of the expectations of (mainly female) employees with family responsibilities, low job satisfaction and limited prospects for intraprofessional development and social mobility.

One of the problems confronting education of nearly all health care professionals is an over-emphasis on factual knowledge, with a relative neglect of interpersonal skills and the ability to synthesize knowledge. While practice-based training fails to provide broader educational and pedagogic support for trainees, course-based training at universities is preparing students insufficiently for their future work. Especially for physicians, practice-based education during their studies is lacking and interdisciplinary work does not form part of their training.

Although there is now a broad consensus that health professionals should be better qualified in primary care, health promotion, rehabilitative care and interdisciplinary work, the majority of trainees are still almost exclusively trained and specialized in secondary or tertiary hospitals for acute care. In November 2002, however, the University of Greifswald established the first Institute for Community-Based Medicine in Germany.

Working conditions

More than one-quarter of the health care workforce (29% in 2003) works part-time, a figure that is significantly above the national average of 15%. A further 9% are "marginally employed", compared to a national average of 13%. There are important gender differences: men in the health sector more frequently work full-time (89.2%) than women (57.1%).

In hospitals the workload has increased in recent years, with a declining average duration of stay and a rising throughput. At the same time, many hospitals have reduced their personnel because of budgetary constraints. Another challenge facing the hospital sector is the organization of inpatient care. Each medical department is led by a relatively autonomous head. As a result, the process of inpatient care is organized around the needs of the individual departments, rather than according to considerations of cost–effectiveness. In addition, few hospital managers have enacted comprehensive human resource strategies that support continuing education and career development.

In ambulatory care, an intensive workload has also become a problem. As the financial allocations from mandatory care insurance have not been adapted to inflation or wage increases, many ambulatory care units remain understaffed and are unable to provide adequate care. For this reason, a number of cases of neglected or mistreated elderly people have been reported in recent years.

According to a survey undertaken in 1998/1999 in five countries, 17.4% of nurses in Germany reported dissatisfaction with their current job and 16.7% were planning to leave their job in the next year, the lowest values of all countries included in the study. Concerning their own competence and their relationship to physicians, nurses in Germany, however, were quite content (Aiken et al. 2001). A more recent study in 10 European countries showed similar results, with 18.5% of nurses in Germany thinking about leaving their jobs, although in this case lower values were found in most other countries included in the study (NEXT study group 2003).

Personnel shortages persist in many parts of the health care system. What seems to be required is a comprehensive system of human resource planning and, in some places, a reduction of the workload. However, the scarcity of resources serves as an impediment to adequate staffing levels. In addition, in September 2001, the European Court of Justice ruled that on-call duty should be considered a part of overall working hours, which was not previously the case in Germany. Although the judgement was suspended for two years, it is expected to result in a considerable increase in personnel costs, as hospitals have to introduce new working schedules and employ more staff.

Performance management

While Germany still lacks a comprehensive monitoring system concerned with the performance of personnel, several important developments relating to ambulatory and hospital care have taken place in recent years.

In order to provide about 30% of the catalogue of ambulatory services (mostly invasive or scanning procedures), providers need to meet certain certification requirements, in addition to being licensed as specialists. These requirements include technical standards, organizational structures and additional training, the latter being defined as a minimum number of procedures undertaken under supervision. The requirements are established by the Federal Association of Physicians.

In the hospital sector, purchasers are allowed to enter into contracts only with hospitals which meet minimum requirements. These requirements, however, are not an indicator of high quality. For a number of services, delivery of a predefined minimum number of procedures is the criterion for being contracted by purchasers and it is highly questionable whether volume alone is an adequate quality indicator.

Nevertheless, more emphasis has been given to quality assurance in recent years. An independent institute for quality assurance has been established and quality of care has become an obligatory component of the contracts between purchasers and providers. So far, the contracts oblige the providers to document the quality of care for a set of surgical procedures (such as hip or cataract surgery) and invasive medical procedures (such as implantation of pacemakers).

Regulation

As already mentioned, in the 1980s, sickness funds and physicians' associations demanded a reduction in the supply of physicians. In the 1990s, the admission of physicians to ambulatory care became more and more restricted. Since 1993, the need for physicians has been calculated on the basis of the regional distribution of physicians in the mandatory health insurance system in 1990. The country has been divided into 10 geographical categories, ranging from large cities to rural areas, and the need per group of physicians was defined as the number of physicians per population that was working in each geographical category in 1990. New practices are not allowed to be opened in areas where supply exceeds 110% of that figure. However, factors such as age, gender, morbidity, mortality, the socioeconomic status of the respective population covered, or the supply of hospital beds, were not taken into account. The defined need for certain specialties varies widely between different geographical categories. The variance is greatest for psychotherapists, for which a norm of one psychotherapist per 2577 population was established in the most urban areas, while in rural areas the corresponding figure was one psychotherapist per 23 106 population.

As mentioned above, the 1993 Health Care Structure Law regulated the number of nurses based on standard nursing times. While this regulation was applied between 1993 and 1996, it has since been discontinued, as it led to an unexpected increase in nursing staffing levels.

Legislation concerning many medical professions was reformed during the 1990s. Some professions, such as psychological psychotherapists, for the first time gained the status of a registered health profession, with far-reaching consequences for their position in the mandatory health insurance system.

The judgement of the European Court of Justice on on-call times is expected to have a significant impact on working conditions, particularly in hospitals. It is likely to increase personnel costs and trigger new working methods, such as working in shifts.

The main challenges faced by decision-makers with regard to the regulation of health professionals relate to the scarcity of resources and increasing demands for qualified personnel and quality services. In the future, it will be necessary to put a greater emphasis on continuing education, and a curriculum that will take account of new information technologies and an ageing population. The health care system will need to learn to manage its workforce more professionally and to improve communication and cooperation between different health professions. Until now, corporatist self-regulation, the hierarchical structure of the workforce, and professional fragmentation have worked as barriers to the implementation of appropriate regulations for the health care workforce.

Conclusions

Human resources in the German health sector are facing a series of demands, both from inside and outside the professions. While personnel shortages persist in some areas, such as care for elderly people, there have been increased budgetary constraints in recent years across the health care sector.

Although human resources are the main productive factor in health care, they are not yet appropriately valued and managed in Germany. It will be essential in the future to establish a comprehensive system of personnel planning, development and management at all levels of the health sector. The medical profession will need to be redefined in order to allow for increased autonomy of the patient, better management of chronic and psychosomatic diseases and increased interdisciplinary networking.

REFERENCES

Advisory Council (2001). *Report 2000/2001.* Bonn, Advisory Council for Concerted Action in Health Care, Federal Ministry of Health.

Aiken L et al. (2001). Nurses' reports on hospital care in five countries. *Health Affairs,* 20: 43–53.

Arnold M, Klauber J, Schnellschmidt H (2002). *Krankenhaus-Report 2001.* Stuttgart, New York, Schattauer Verlag.

Arnold M, Klauber J, Schnellschmidt H (2003). *Krankenhaus-Report 2002.* Stuttgart, New York, Schattauer Verlag.

Federal Statistical Office (2003a). *Gesundheit, Personal 1997–2002.* Wiesbaden, Federal Statistical Office.

Federal Statistical Office (2003b). *Statistical yearbook, health.* Wiesbaden, Federal Statistical Office.

Federal Statistical Office (2005). *Statistical yearbook, health.* Wiesbaden, Federal Statistical Office.

Kälble K (2002). Entwicklung der Studiengänge im Bereich Gesundheit. In: Klüsche W, ed. *Entwicklung von Studium und Praxis in den Sozial- und Gesundheitsberufen.* Mönchengladbach, Hochschule Niederrhein (Schriften des Fachbereichs Sozialwesen der Hochschule Niederrhein, Volume 24).

Kälble K (2003). Strukturen der Weiterbildung und die Einführung von Bachelor und Masterprogrammen an deutschen Hochschulen – Ein Beitrag zur Herstellung von Transparenz und Orientierung hinsichtlich ökonomie- und managementorientierter Bildungsangebote für Ärztinnen und Ärzte. In: Burk R, Hellman W, eds. *Krankenhausmanagement für Ärztinnen und Ärzte.* Berlin, Ecomed Verlag KVB.

Kassenärztliche Bundesvereinigung (2001). *Grunddaten zur vertragsärztlichen Versorgung in Deutschand. Berlin,* Kassenärztliche Bundesvereinigung (http://daris.kbv.de/daris/link. asp?ID=1003739521).

Kassenärztliche Bundesvereinigung (2002). *Die ärztliche Versorgung in der Bundesrepublik Deutschland am 31.12.2001.* Cologne, Deutscher Ärzte-Verlag *(Blaue Reihe No. 54).*

NEXT-study group (2003). *The European NEXT-study.* Wuppertal, University of Wuppertal (http://www.next.uni-wuppertal.de/download/BrochurePRESSTNEXTEN2005.pdf).

OECD (2004). *Health data 2004.* Paris, Organisation for Economic Co-operation and Development (http://www.oecd.org).

OECD (2005). *Health data 2005.* Paris, Organisation for Economic Co-operation and Development (http://www.oecd.org).

WHO (2005). European Health for All database (HFA-DB) [online database], Copenhagen, WHO Regional Office for Europe.

Chapter 4
Lithuania

Žilvinas Padaiga, Liudvika Starkienė, Zeneta Logminiene, Jack Reamy

Setting the context

During the period of Soviet occupation, Lithuania operated the Semashko model that existed throughout the Soviet Union. The health system was centralized, with facilities owned and managed by the state, and health personnel were government employees. The focus was on the quantity of hospitals and physicians rather than on primary care services or the quality of care provided.

Since 1990, when Lithuania declared independence, the health system has undergone substantial reforms that aimed to improve population health, address issues of equity, establish consumer choice and improve the quality of care. A major element of the health care reforms was an increased focus on primary health care and the introduction of general practitioners.

In the area of health financing, a statutory health insurance system has been introduced progressively since 1997, establishing a split between providers and purchasers of health services. The national Health Insurance Fund, accountable to the Ministry of Health, is now responsible for the allocation and distribution of resources. The health insurance system is financed by a combination of insurance contributions and, predominantly, tax revenues.

There were also changes in the ownership of health facilities, with decentralization of the organizational structure of the health system. Most health facilities have been transformed into non-profit-making enterprises. The 10 counties and 60 municipalities of the country have assumed authority over health facilities on their territories. The counties manage county hospitals and tertiary care facilities, while municipalities are responsible for the provision of primary health care and public health activities. The Ministry of Health is in charge of the overall regulation and organization of the health system. Two parallel health systems are run by the Ministry of Internal Affairs and the Ministry of Defence (Centre for Health Economics 2000; Cerniauskas and Murauskiene 2000; Lovkyte et al. 2003).

Major problems facing the Lithuanian health care system are the lack of funds for the health sector and the continued orientation of health services towards specialized and hospital services. An additional problem is ageing, with a decreasing percentage of the population being of working age. The national health policy aims to shift resources from hospitals to primary care providers, retrain more physicians to become general practitioners and to restructure some hospitals towards more nurse-oriented institutions.

Workforce supply

According to the National Statistical Department, in 2001, 7% of the total workforce in Lithuania was employed in the health sector, an increase from 5.6% in 1992. 18% of the health care workforce were physicians. Currently, however, precise data on active human resources in the health sector are lacking (Gaizauskiene et al. 2003). The Lithuanian Health Information Centre has provided annual data on the number of physicians since 1993. It collects information on the number of physical persons and full-time equivalents and on the distribution in terms of regions and specialties.

A comprehensive system for the planning of human resources in the health sector has so far been lacking. There is no legal document regulating human resource planning in Lithuania and there was no consistent policy in dealing with geographical imbalances in the distribution of human resources (WHO 2001).

Physicians

Planning of the number of physicians in the health sector has not been a high priority in the last decade and there continues to be an oversupply. Lithuania traditionally had a large number of hospital beds per capita and one of the highest numbers of physicians per population in Europe. The relative number of physicians has remained remarkably stable since independence. The ratio of physicians to population was 410 per 100 000 people in 1992, decreasing slightly to 398 in 2002. The largest percentage of physicians (46.5%) was between 36 and 50 years of age and 15% of physicians were older than 60

(Gaizauskiene et al. 2003; Lovkyte et al. 2003; National Statistical Department 2003).

The largest proportion of physicians in 2000 were specialists in internal medicine (31%), with smaller numbers in paediatrics (14%), surgery (6%) and obstetrics and gynaecology (6%). As a result of primary health care reforms, the number of general practitioners has increased almost nine times since 1993.

There has traditionally been a strong female representation among physicians. In 2000, 69% of physicians were women, with the largest proportion among paediatricians (92%) and general practitioners (85%). The only specialties with a minority of female physicians were surgery (9%), orthopaedic surgery (11%), forensic medicine (18%) and paediatric surgery (34%). The share of women in the physician workforce is set to increase further. At Kaunas University of Medicine, the share of women among enrolled medical students increased from 65% in 1995 to 82% in 2001 (Gaizauskiene et al. 2003; Lovkyte et al. 2003).

The geographical distribution of physicians is uneven, with the majority working in urban areas. In 2002, 614 physicians per 100 000 population were working in urban areas, compared to 242 per 100 000 in rural areas. There was also an uneven distribution across counties. In 2002, Vilnius and Kaunas counties, hosting the country's medical faculties and tertiary care university hospitals, had an average of 518 physicians per 100 000 population, while the remaining eight counties had on average 288 physicians per 100 000 population (Lithuanian Health Information Centre 2003; Lovkyte et al. 2003).

In a survey in 2002, 60.7% of specialist trainees and 26.8% of physicians taking part in the study expressed their intention to leave Lithuania. It can be expected that EU accession has facilitated the emigration of physicians and nurses, although precise data on the number of health care workers who have emigrated are not available.

Managers of health institutions are generally physicians. So far, there is no system for the training of health managers and the training of some physicians as health administrators is not sufficient to fill this gap.

Nurses

The last decade has seen a reduction of nurses in both absolute and relative numbers, similar to developments in other countries of central and eastern Europe. The absolute number of nurses decreased from 30 080 in 1990 to 28 120 in 1998, while the number of midwives decreased from 3970 to 1610.

In relative terms, the number of nurses decreased from 1098 per 100 000 population in 1990 to 777 in 2002 (Lithuanian Health Information Centre 2003). In 2003, there were 27 787 nurses working in the health sector, 99.5% of whom were women (WHO 2005). Most nurses work in the inpatient sector. However, the recently enacted Law on Nursing Practice, which legalized community nursing, may encourage employment in the primary care sector.

A dramatic decline has occurred in terms of nursing graduates in the last decade. In 1991, 49.43 nurses graduated per 100 000 population, a ratio that had decreased to 5.48 in 1999. The ratio of graduate physicians to graduate nurses decreased from 1 to 4.7 in 1991 to 1 to 0.6 in 1999. The decline in numbers of graduate nurses is likely to be related to the profession's low prestige and salary.

The decrease in the number of employed nurses was triggered by the health reform process. It was easier for health institutions to dismiss nurses than doctors, while the economic gain was similar, as there are no major differences in salaries. In addition, trade unions representing nurses are still comparatively weak. These trends in the employment and graduation of nurses are particularly worrying, as there is likely to be an increasing demand for nurses in the future, owing in part to the ageing of the Lithuanian population as well as to a shift in professional demarcation.

As is the case with physicians, the geographical distribution of nurses in the country is very uneven. According to data from the Lithuanian Health Information Centre, in 2002, the number of nurses in urban areas was 970 per 100 000 population, compared to 572 in rural areas (Lithuanian Health Information Centre 2003). The Ministry of Health has tried to attract health care workers to rural areas through financial incentives, but these have been too low to result in substantial changes in the regional distribution of nurses.

Education and training

Since independence, medical education has undergone substantial reforms. Following EU requirements and WHO recommendations, postgraduate training was introduced and undergraduate education reformed.

Physicians

Physicians are trained at the medical faculty of Vilnius University and at Kaunas University of Medicine. Education of health professionals is state-financed. However, in addition to a defined number of places, students may gain entry to medical studies by paying the full study costs themselves.

For admission to medical studies, completed secondary education is required. Admission is based on the results of final school examinations and average school marks. Foreign citizens and persons without citizenship are required to pass an entrance examination. About 15% of medical students drop out of their studies. Medical studies are assessed using practical and theoretical state examinations. After completion of six years of medical studies, graduates receive a diploma. In 2003, the Ministry of Health, in conjunction with the Ministry of Education and Science, determined the minimum requirements for the training of physicians, dentists, pharmacists, nurses and midwives.

The number of state-financed students admitted to medical studies is determined by the universities with medical faculties, in conjunction with the Ministry of Health, the Ministry of Education and the Ministry of Finance. In 1994, this number was set at 240 students, with additional places for students paying the full study costs. In the years between 1989 and 1999, the number of state-financed students was reduced by 30%. A project group for planning of human resources in health was created in 2000, projecting that the supply of physicians would decrease by 25% by 2015 if the enrolment of students remained at the level of 250 students per year. Starting in 2002, the number of study places was increased to 400 students per year (Gaizauskiene et al. 2003).

A system of postgraduate specialization based on residencies was introduced in 1992. The duration of the specialization varies from three years (such as for family medicine and ophthalmology) to six years (such as for paediatric cardiology and paediatric neurology). The theoretical part of the training is taught at the country's two medical faculties, while the practical part includes training at clinical sites under supervision of a practising physician. The salaries for residents and their trainers is paid by the universities. The number of specialties financed from the state budget was set at 110 in 1993. Currently, there are 18 medical specialties for physicians. Specialists in family medicine are either trained in residencies or in retraining programmes with the same content and requirements.

Practising physicians are required to renew their licences every five years. For this purpose, they are required to collect at least 200 credit hours of continuing medical education. At least 60% of these credits must be obtained from universities, while the remaining credits can be accrued in training provided by professional associations. The Ministry of Health is responsible for establishing standards in continuing medical education and partly finances it. Physicians in the public sector are given paid leave for attending continuing medical education.

Nurses

In the Soviet period, nurses were educated in two-year diploma training programmes in so-called "medical schools" outside universities. Medical schools were institutions for the technical training of allied health professionals. The teachers mostly comprised physicians. To enter nursing training, secondary education was not required. While for practising nurses, continuing medical education was not mandatory, they were offered specialization, based on one to six months of additional coursework.

One of the most fundamental reforms of the training of health care workers after independence was the introduction of university education for nursing. In 1990, the first Faculty of Nursing was established at Kaunas University of Medicine. In 1996, study programmes for nurses were offered for students who had completed secondary education.

Students of nursing can pursue a bachelor's degree in nursing science, which takes three academic years for students who have attended college and four years for students without college education. University-based studies are offered at the nursing faculty at Kaunas University of Medicine, at the medical faculty of Vilnius University and at Klaipeda University. Part-time studies for working nurses are offered at Kaunas University of Medicine and at Klaipeda University. In 1994, a master's degree in nursing for graduates with bachelor's degrees was introduced and is now offered at five universities in Lithuania. In the period between 1994 and 2002, about 30% of nurses who had completed undergraduate studies continued their education in master's programmes, with the percentage increasing over time. Those who wish to continue their university education can then embark on four years of doctoral studies, a possibility which was introduced in 1999. Nurses with postgraduate education generally work in the upper levels of health administration, in positions such as nursing directors or clinical administrators.

The curriculum of nursing studies has been revised to include health promotion and community care. There is also an increased emphasis on practical skills and the involvement of qualified nurses in the training programme. At the beginning of the reform of nursing education in Lithuania, trainers were invited from abroad, mainly from the Nordic countries, helping to train a first group of trainers. A large part of the first cohort of graduate nursing students remained at the universities and became lecturers.

In 2000, a survey of the nursing teaching personnel was conducted. The results were surprising. Only 39% of respondents felt that nurses should be able to make decisions independently, only 26.4% thought that nursing training should develop analytical and critical thinking, while only 7.5% found it necessary for nurses to acquire organizational abilities. The respondents saw nurses not as independent professionals, but primarily as persons implementing the orders of physicians (Zydziunaite 2002).

At present, much attention is being devoted to expanding training in nursing administration. 80% of nurses completing bachelor's degrees choose a career in the administration of nursing. Nursing management and administration have recently been included in the regular curricula of undergraduate nursing studies and in the continuing education of nurses.

The system of continuing education has been reorganized in the last decade. In 1994, the Training and Specialization Centre for Nurses was established, responsible for the continuing education and retraining of nurses. In 1998, 14 861 nurses participated in courses provided by the centre. Nurses educated in the old educational system are required to undergo a retraining course offered by the centre. Courses of continuing education and retraining are financed to a level of 75% by the Ministry of Health. The remaining 25% has to be paid by the employers or trainees. Owing to limited resources, there are at present more applicants for courses than the centre can admit (Ruolia 2001).

In addition to the training of nurses in universities, there continues to be nursing training outside universities, currently provided by six colleges. The duration of the training has been extended to three and a half years, but has still been found to fall short of EU requirements.

The Law on Nursing Practice sets out the legal basis for nursing and the rights and duties of nurses. It envisages the licensing and certification of nurses. Those nurses with a university education have the right to receive a licence to practise as a general nurse. Nurses trained in colleges can also apply for the licence, provided they have at least three years of work experience in the last five years and have received at least 100 hours of professional education during this period. Once nurses have been issued with a licence, they are required to extend its validity every five years. General nurses have been required to have licences to practise since October 2003, while specialized nurses have required a special licence since October 2005.

Although major efforts to reform nursing education have been made in Lithuania in recent years, there continue to be a number of challenges, including the lack of financial and human resources, a lack of support from the Ministry of Health and health care institutions, and a lack of initiative among the nursing profession.

Health managers

Vilnius University and Kaunas University of Medicine have started to offer training courses for health managers. A programme for a master's degree in public health management was introduced in 2000 at Kaunas University of Medicine. The course takes two years on a full-time and three years on a part-time basis. The studies have to be financed by the students themselves or third-party funders.

Working conditions

In the period following independence, the health sector suffered less from unemployment than other sectors of society. According to labour force surveys, fewer than 4700 health care workers have lost their jobs since 1993. The vast majority of them were female auxiliaries in urban areas. In 2002, about 1000 nurses were unemployed, compared to 27 787 employed nurses (National Statistical Department 2003).

Salaries of health care professionals working in the public sector have traditionally been low and amounted to 83% of the national average in 1999. Since 1996, however, wages in the health sector have increased more than the national average. One reason for the low salaries in the health sector may be the dominance of female employees. In other sectors of the Lithuanian economy, women receive on average about 80% of what their male counterparts earn, despite legal guarantees of non-discrimination. In 2000, physicians received on average €260 per month, with significantly higher average salaries for male physicians (€296) than for females (€246) (Centre for Health Economics 2000).

Although there are some exceptions, the salaries of health care workers in Lithuanian health facilities are generally not linked to any kind of incentives that would enhance productivity or the quality of work. The statutory salaries of the main professional groups are financed from the health insurance fund. Since 1991, public health institutions have been allowed to introduce internal payment systems based on elements of fee-for-service or capitation, within the framework of collective bargaining and the legal minimum wage. However, even in those institutions that have introduced these elements, regular salaries account for about 70% of the income of physicians (Cerniauskas and Murauskiene 2000).

Up to 90% of physicians are working in public hospitals and polyclinics and are paid regular salaries. General practitioners, paediatricians, gynaecologists, surgeons and psychiatrists who work in rural areas are paid an additional allowance of €27 per month. Primary health care physicians are paid on a capitation basis, with adjustments for the age and geographical distribution of the population covered. These payments cover all recurrent costs of services, offering little incentive to increase productivity (Cerniauskas and Murauskiene 2000). The minimum and maximum size of the population serviced by a primary health care specialist was determined in 2000. Reimbursement of secondary and tertiary care providers is based on a price list for services.

The working week of health care personnel was set at 39 hours in 1997. Since 2001, the heads of health care institutions have determined the working hours of their staff. The workload of physicians was determined in 1994. In outpatient polyclinics, the workload was calculated according to the number of patient and home visits. In inpatient facilities, the workload was established on the basis of the number of patients served per physician.

As mentioned above, there was a decrease in the number of employed nurses. With the aim of avoiding further dismissals, the Ministry of Health issued an order in 1997, stipulating the proportion of the salary funds of health institutions that should be allocated to nurses. In polyclinics and primary care centres, this proportion was set at 40%, while in nursing hospitals it was set at 60%.

According to a survey conducted in Lithuania in 1995, nurses mainly focused on technical tasks not directly centred on patients. At present, the workload of nurses is not described in any legal documents, except for nurses working in intensive care units, where a nurse is required for every two patients. Nurses working in tertiary care institutions and in urban areas tend to be younger and better educated. In more rural areas, the workload of nurses is smaller, but they provide a broader spectrum of services, including social work, community nursing, home nursing and also unskilled work such as cleaning.

Overall, staff turnover and mobility of nurses are minimal. The career structure depends on the size and character of the health care institution. For nurses without a university education, career possibilities are very limited. The positions of head nurses are mainly reserved for nurses with a university education. The university-based training has in general opened new career possibilities for nurses, as they can now pursue scientific, pedagogical or administrative careers. However, nurses with a university education often encounter opposition by head nurses educated in the Soviet system. In addition, nursing studies are more up to date than medical studies, so that nurses face some opposition from physicians when applying their knowledge.

Two professional associations for nurses have emerged since independence. In 1992, the Lithuanian Nursing Organization was founded and several years later the University Nursing Society. Both organizations aim to represent and protect the rights of Lithuanian nurses. The Lithuanian Nursing Organization currently counts about 45% of Lithuania's nurses as its members. It actively participates in the adoption of legal documents relating to nurses. The organization, however, has limited political influence, mainly because of the low prestige of the nursing profession.

Performance management

As mentioned above, the wages of health care personnel are generally fixed and financial incentives to improve performance are therefore lacking. Non-financial tools for the encouragement of performance are not widely used in Lithuania's health system.

The performance of health care workers and the quality of services provided are primarily regulated by licensing and certification, which are described in the following section. An internal medical audit system in health care institutions was started in 1998. It aims to ensure the quality of services provided. In addition, physicians and nurses are required to improve their qualifications through continuing education.

Regulation

The National Board of Health is responsible for the coordination of health policy in Lithuania, which is implemented by the Ministry of Health. The ministry is mainly a coordinating and regulating body. In conjunction with other relevant ministries or institutions, it coordinates and regulates education and training, licensing and certification, working conditions and performance standards. The ministry is also, at least formally, responsible for the planning of human resources in the health sector.

Licensing and accreditation of public and private health care institutions is carried out by the State Accreditation Agency under the Ministry of Health.

The Medical Audit Inspectorate under the Ministry of Health, established in 1998, is involved in the establishment of medical standards and quality control with respect to health care providers. Until 1996, when the Law on Medical Practice was adopted, the medical practice of physicians was not legally defined. In the period between 1995 and 2001, the Ministry of Health, in conjunction with the Ministry of Education, the universities and the professional organizations, prepared and approved medical standards for different categories of physicians and nurses. Guidelines on nursing services have also been established by the Lithuanian Nursing Organization. They have not been approved by the Ministry of Health, but have been adopted by some health care institutions. There are also health care providers that have introduced information systems documenting nursing care. Professional associations of physicians, nurses, dentists, pharmacists and public health specialists deal with professional standards and the continuing education of their members.

Licensing of health professionals was initiated in 1998, following the Law on Medical Practice of 1996. In connection with the licensing process, a complete register of health care professionals is being developed. The State Accreditation Agency is responsible for the licensing and certification of health care professionals in both the public and private sector. Licences and certificates are issued for a period of five years. Specialists wishing to practise require a certificate from the Ministry of Health.

Conclusions

Since Lithuania gained independence, there have been substantial changes with regard to human resources in the health sector. In the area of medical education, undergraduate studies have been reformed and a system of post-graduate education has been introduced, with physicians specializing during residencies. While medical education has been reorganized, Lithuania traditionally had one of the highest numbers of physicians in Europe, and there continues to be an oversupply of physicians and hospital beds. It remains to be seen whether EU accession will result in major migratory movements of health care workers.

The training of nurses has also undergone far-reaching changes. Nursing studies have been introduced at universities and it is now possible to pursue master's and PhD degrees in nursing. This has increased the prestige of the profession enormously. Increasingly, nurses are being recognized as independent health professionals. It will now be important to formalize this greater recognition. At present, nurses have no representation at the governmental level and leadership positions in the health sector are generally occupied by physicians. There are also challenges relating to quality assurance in nursing. So far, this is not well developed and the working conditions of nurses do not encourage improvement in the quality of services.

It is very likely that Lithuania will soon experience a dramatic shortage of nurses. The number of nursing students has decreased significantly in recent years, while the demand for nurses is expected to increase. One of the main challenges for the future will be the establishment of a comprehensive system of human resource planning. So far, a consistent and long-term policy in this area has been lacking, which will result in serious imbalances between the supply and demand for health care professionals.

Acknowledgement

The authors would like to express their gratitude for support and help provided by the president of the University Nursing Society, Olga Riklikienė.

REFERENCES

Centre for Health Economics (2000). *The first decade of reforms: health care sector in the context of socioeconomic changes* [in Lithuanian]. Vilnius, Centre for Health Economics.

Cerniauskas G, Murauskiene L (2000). *Health care systems in transition: Lithuania.* Copenhagen, WHO Regional Office for Europe, on behalf of the European Observatory on Health Care Systems.

Gaizauskiene A et al. (2003). *Physician planning in Lithuania in 1990–2015.* Kaunas, Open Society Fund.

Lithuanian Health Information Centre (2003). *Population health and activities of health care facilities in Lithuania* [in Lithuanian]. Vilnius, Lithuanian Health Information Centre, Ministry of Health.

Lovkyte L, Reamy J, Padaiga Z (2003). Physicians' resources in Lithuania: change comes slowly. *Croatian Medical Journal,* 44(2): 207–213.

National Statistical Department (2003). *Statistical yearbook of Lithuania 2003.* Vilnius, National Statistical Department.

Ruolia J (2001) Training and specialization centre for nurses, Slauga [in Lithuanian]. *Mokslas ir praktika,* 5(6–7).

WHO (2001). *Highlights on health in Lithuania.* Copenhagen, WHO Regional Office for Europe.

WHO (2005). European Health for All database (HFA-DB) [online database]. Copenhagen, WHO Regional Office for Europe.

Zydziunaite V (2002) Professional nursing education: a prerequisite to acquire nursing qualifications, Slauga [in Lithuanian]. *Mokslas ir praktika,* 35: 10–13.

Chapter 5
Malta

Natasha Azzopardi Muscat, Kenneth Grech

Context

Malta's size and geographical isolation present a unique set of challenges for policy-makers seeking to ensure the provision of comprehensive health services of a high standard. One of the greatest of these challenges is the recruitment, training and retention of highly skilled health care professionals.

Between 1800 and 1964, Malta was a colony of the British Empire. During this period, human resource policies and the training and regulation of health professionals were organized in the same manner as in the United Kingdom. Doctors pursuing a specialization spent a number of years training in the United Kingdom. Those returning to Malta practised in the one and only tertiary hospital. Even after independence, the links between Malta and the United Kingdom remain strong and many health professionals undertake some time of their training there.

In May 2004, Malta acceded to the European Union (EU). This has been the most important factor shaping human resources in health in recent years. The EU employment policies which have been introduced in Malta include the introduction of an additional week of maternity leave and the prohibition of night work for pregnant women. Adoption of the EU Working Time Directive has represented a formidable challenge, as it restricts the total working time per week.

The relationship between politicians and health care workers, particularly doctors, has been a delicate one, as a result of two landmark industrial disputes (German 1991). The first, in the 1950s, occurred when the Government sought to establish a national health service comparable to the one introduced in the United Kingdom in 1948. The medical profession successfully resisted this change and succeeded in establishing the Medical Council of Malta, a regulatory body that allowed a considerable degree of professional self-regulation. The second industrial dispute, lasting from 1977 to 1987, occurred after the Government forced new medical graduates to work for two years in the public sector, a provision which is still in force. The trade union called for a strike, but those doctors who followed this call were "locked out" and were also prohibited from practising in private hospitals. A number of them had no option but to migrate, mostly to the Middle East, and the Government hurriedly imported doctors from elsewhere, mainly from the countries of central and eastern Europe, few of whom could communicate proficiently in English, let alone Maltese. The divisive atmosphere persisted even after the dispute was resolved in 1987, but has now been overcome (Azzopardi Muscat and Dixon 1999).

In macroeconomic terms, Malta is currently experiencing slow economic growth and a high budget deficit, which increase pressures on public sector spending in the context of meeting the convergence criteria for entry to the euro. The constraint on financial resources has acted as a brake on the development of human resource initiatives.

Over 90% of Malta's population are Roman Catholics and traditional values continue to play a major role. Divorce and abortion are illegal. Of the 2004 EU accession countries, Malta had the lowest female participation in the labour force, with only one-third of women in full-time employment (National Statistical Office 2004). Demographically, the country is facing an ageing population. An additional challenge is the brain drain resulting from the emigration of young professionals to other countries.

In the health sector, institutional reforms are still in the making. The national health policy elaborated in 1995, entitled Health Vision 2000, envisaged the establishment of a purchaser–provider split between the Ministry of Health on the one hand and hospitals and health centres on the other, the latter gaining managerial autonomy. However, this policy has not been fully implemented so far. Yet, in January 2004, the tertiary hospital started to achieve managerial autonomy and in the psychiatric hospital nursing officers were given responsibility for managing the resources allocated to their wards.

Workforce supply

The total number of physicians listed in the registers of the Medical Council in 2003 was 1285, equivalent to 321 per 100 000 population. The European Health for All database lists 291 per 100 000 population, which is based on the principal list, recording all medical graduates from the University of Malta.

The number of physicians in Malta has continuously increased in recent years, in particular the number of female physicians, constituting 35.2% of medical practitioners registered with the Medical Council in 2004. The registers of the Medical Council, however, tend to overestimate the supply of physicians in the country, as they do not take account of inactive physicians or physicians migrating abroad. Although precise data are lacking, it can be estimated that 70–80% of medical graduates migrate, mainly to the United Kingdom and the United States. A considerable proportion of those who specialize abroad do not return to Malta. EU accession appears to be further facilitating this process (Azzopardi Muscat 2002). With regard to the inflow of workers from the European Economic Area (EEA), Malta has negotiated a seven-year period with the EU, during which it may restrict immigration if serious imbalances occur. This regulation, however, does not apply to self-employed professionals.

Until very recently, the Medical Council has not kept registers for specialists, so that there are no precise data on the number of specialists in contrast to generalists. In primary care, most doctors work full-time in the private sector, with twice as many patient contacts in the private as in the public sector (MoH 2003). Nearly all physicians employed in public hospitals also work in the private sector, compensating for poor salaries in the public sector. About 500 doctors work in the country's five main public hospitals and 84 in the public primary health care sector. Of the doctors working in hospitals, 28% are women. Although more female doctors now graduate, few manage to specialize and reach higher levels of clinical responsibility. The career paths of women are especially affected by their role in child care (Melillo 2001). A project supported by the European Social Fund aims to improve representation of women at senior clinical and management levels.

Accurate data on the number of nurses are not readily available, as the registers of the Council for Nurses and Midwives do not regularly remove deceased persons. According to data from the Directorate of Nursing Services, at the end of 2003, 1746 nurses were employed in the public health sector, equivalent to 435 nurses per 100 000 population. While "enrolled nurses" (nurses with generally lower levels of school education who have not been trained in universities) still outnumber "state-registered nurses", courses for enrolled nurses have now ceased and upgrading courses for enrolled nurses are being provided. Nursing specialties have only started to be developed very recently. Migration of nurses is the exception rather than the rule and the number of nurses going abroad remains negligible. There has been a small-scale immigration of nurses from the former Yugoslavia and developing countries. Only once, in the early 1990s, were 50 nurses actively recruited from the United Kingdom and most have now left Malta.

Health managers are usually doctors or nurses who have specialized in health services management or who occupy management positions as a result of their seniority in the system. Historically, health managers emerged from among the clinical staff. The nursing profession is led hierarchically by middle and senior nursing managers and other clinical professions are organized along the same lines. Each hospital doctor works within a unit led by a consultant, who holds overall clinical responsibility. In addition, physicians are organized in clinical departments headed by chairpersons chosen from among the consultants. Hospital management is generally in the hands of medical administrators or superintendents. In recent years, nonmedical personnel have taken over some of the management positions in hospitals. While the Institute of Health Care has been offering courses in health services management since the late 1990s, none of the current clinical directors has undergone management training.

Paramedical professions face many of the same issues as nurses. Migration has not played a major role and there is a significant number of women with family responsibilities. None of the paramedical professions are licensed to practise independently, although some nurses and paramedics do so informally. Following the creation of the Institute of Health Care, the supply of paramedical professionals increased rapidly in the 1990s. None of the courses has a *numerus clausus*, apart from physiotherapy.

Dentistry is mostly a private sector activity, as the public health service only covers certain population groups and emergency treatment. Pharmacists are also mainly employed in the private sector, where they mostly work in community retail pharmacies and as medical representatives of pharmaceutical companies. While a *numerus clausus* is required for the study of dentistry, no restriction exists with regard to the number of pharmacy students.

One of the main challenges associated with the workforce supply is the establishment of live databases on the health care workforce. Another challenge is the chronic shortage of doctors in the public primary health care sector. Many doctors have left this area in recent years, owing to low pay, restricted opportunities for training or career progression and poor working conditions (Sammut 2003). An additional reason why few doctors are attracted by primary health care is that it is not given sufficient importance in undergraduate medical studies. There is also a shortage of junior doctors pursuing internships, temporarily alleviated each time a fresh cohort of doctors completes their studies. In some medical specialties, on the other hand, there is an oversupply, as only one specialist hospital exists in the country. In the next few years there may also be an oversupply in some paramedical professions, such as radiography and medical laboratory science. In general, it is very difficult to move staff between departments and institutions, as the trade unions fiercely resist staff redeployment.

For the past few years, the Health Division of the Ministry of Health has had a workforce plan. The plan provided young health care professionals with useful information on the planned growth in specialist areas. One of the most successful strategies in redressing imbalances in the workforce supply was pursued in the late 1980s and early 1990s, aiming to overcome a severe nursing shortage. The strategy tried to attract students to nursing, retain nurses in employment, and entice female nurses back to the profession. Nursing education was upgraded to courses leading to a certificate, diploma or bachelor's degree. For working nurses, a series of incentives were introduced, including a marked increase in salary and status. A 60-bed geriatric rehabilitation hospital was entirely staffed by nurses returning to work, who were attracted by retraining courses, flexible working hours and a child care centre. As part of the planning process for a new general hospital, it is envisaged that a comprehensive workforce plan for the whole health sector be set up.

Education and training

Malta boasts one of the oldest universities and medical schools in Europe. The University of Malta traces its origins to the founding of the Collegium Melitense in 1592, while medical undergraduate training was established in 1676. Today, medical studies consist of five years of formal training at university, plus at least one year of supervised practice. The first two years of studies are pre-clinical, the last three clinical. In the late 1980s and early 1990s, the University of Malta opened its doors to all students with the qualification for admission to university. The *numerus clausus* for medical studies was formally lifted in 1998. The Ministry of Health does not formally regulate the number of students enrolled or the quality and content of the teaching programmes. However, an expert group appointed by the European Commission which examined course outlines and modules in 2002 found them in conformity with EU requirements.

In 2003, 37 students graduated from medical courses (24 male and 13 female), 13 students from the dentistry course (6 male and 7 female) and 24 from the pharmacy course (7 male and 17 female). The medical and dental faculties are financed by the Ministry of Education. There are no fees for undergraduate education and students are paid a stipend for their studies by the Government. The University of Malta employs teaching staff, although only a handful of physicians are dedicated to teaching on a full-time basis and most work full-time in clinical positions and have been attracted to lecturing positions by honorary posts. The partnership of units with similar organizations abroad has helped to improve the quality of teaching and provide mobility to students. One of the biggest problems faced by teaching staff is that student numbers have increased, while teaching staff has not. Low salaries and limited learning and teaching resources act as barriers to attracting professionals to the university on a full-time basis.

All health professionals have to follow the same educational pathway to enter university. After primary and secondary school between 5 and 16 years of age, pupils are required to attend the Junior College of the university or a private school for two years, in order to obtain the qualification for admission to university. However, each university course has slightly different entry requirements, with regard to the marks achieved in various subjects. The most stringent requirements exist for medical and dental courses.

In recent years, there has been much progress in continuing professional development and the establishment of postgraduate and specialist training. In contrast to undergraduate education, most postgraduate education comes at a cost. In addition, training physicians have to pay for their exams at foreign institutions, such as colleges in the United Kingdom. For the past 15 years, the faculties for medicine and dentistry have offered MPhil and PhD programmes. In several areas, doctors can now obtain their entire specialist training in Malta. Complex specialized services, such as cardiac surgery and heart or lung transplantation, have been established, reducing Malta's dependency on centres abroad. The main challenge now is to formalize the training content and procedures. The specialty of public health has grown rapidly since 1995, when the first programme for a master's degree in public health was organized by the University of Malta. Since 2001, the course has also been open to non-medical professionals. A new programme has been devised for vocational training for general practitioners.

While continuing medical education has gained importance in recent years, it is still not obligatory. The activities in this area are mainly organized by the professional organizations and funded by the pharmaceutical industry or other health-related companies. However, doctors, dentists and pharmacists can claim a fixed sum (€1200) per year for continuing professional development, an entitlement nursing and paramedical professionals do not yet have.

Recent years have also seen an increase in the number of doctors undergoing the new health services management courses. Health professionals are also increasingly attending courses for master's degrees in management or for a Master of Business Administration.

Formal undergraduate teaching of nurses and allied professions is a more recent phenomenon. The School of Nursing was established by the Ministry of Health in the 1960s and courses for other health professions commenced in the 1980s. The Institute of Health Care was set up within the University of Malta in 1992, replacing the School of Nursing which was part of the Ministry of Health and fully funded by it. This change was the most important institutional reform of the education of health care professionals in recent years, and raised the status of nursing education. The Institute of Health Care provides both diploma and master's courses in nursing and in a number of paramedical professions. The institute is subsidized by the Ministry of Health, which is represented on its managing board.

The teaching of nurses has been upgraded from a certificate to a degree course. Many nurses have undergone courses to upgrade their qualifications from the status of an enrolled nurse, signified by a certificate, to a state-registered nurse, which is the nursing qualification recognized throughout Europe. In addition, nurses have started to obtain postgraduate qualifications.

All health professionals qualifying from the University of Malta and, since May 2004, from universities of the European Economic Area are automatically eligible for registration with the relevant professional body. Some professions, namely doctors, dentists, midwives and pharmacists, are additionally issued with a licence from the President of Malta, marking the professions allowed to practise independently. Certification is used as the mechanism for awarding specialist status. To date, specialist accreditation committees have been set up for medicine and dentistry.

One of the challenges associated with the education of health professionals will be to overcome the distinction between medical faculties and the Institute of Health Care, which are at present totally separate institutions. There are long-term plans for the creation of a single Institute of Health Sciences, but at present the two teaching cultures are still very disparate.

Working conditions

All employees in the public health care sector are directly employed by the Government and form part of the civil service. Health professionals enter the civil service quasi-automatically after graduation and a university degree has traditionally been viewed as a guarantee of a safe job. While doctors, dentists and pharmacists can enter the service at any level, nurses and other allied professionals can only enter at the lowest possible salary level, irrespective of their qualification and experience. The public health care sector currently employs over 5000 clinical and non-clinical staff. Another 1500 professionals work in the field of social care. While official data are not available, the large private sector has experienced unprecedented growth in recent years.

Private general practitioners form the backbone of family medicine in Malta, accounting for over 60% of all general practitioners working in the community. The vast majority of them work in single practices. Public sector doctors and nurses in the primary care sector are subject to the same conditions as hospital employees.

As part of wide-ranging reforms throughout the civil service, conditions of employment have improved significantly in recent years. These improvements include family-friendly measures, such as the right to a career break of three years after the birth of every child, in addition to one year of unpaid leave. The introduction of the EU Working Time Directive has had an effect on the working hours and schedules of specialists and doctors in training. At present, doctors, many of whom work up to 50–60 hours per week, have opted out of the directive. The revision of the directive is a sensitive and important area for Malta. Should the possibility to opt out be removed, Malta could need twice as many specialists at senior registrar level.

Physicians working in the public sector receive basic salaries ranging from €15 000–20 000 per year for doctors and €25 000 for consultants. Many doctors, other than consultants, however, double their earnings by working longer than the regular 40-hour week. Physicians in the private sector are paid on a fee-for-service basis.

A comprehensive workforce plan is in place for doctors in the public health care sector. In accordance with this plan, the Government periodically issues calls for applications for training posts in various specialties. It is still common, however, for Maltese doctors to spend between two and five years abroad. On completion of their training, doctors are eligible for senior positions at either senior registrar or consultant level.

Like physicians, following their graduation, nurses are usually employed by the Government. Nurses can expect to earn €15 000–27 000 for a working week of 46.6 hours. They rely on the supplementation of their basic salaries through extra allowances, for example for working in shifts, at night or on Sundays. To date, promotions are based on years of experience rather than on qualifications or aptitude.

Most paramedical professionals have a working week of 40 hours in 6 days, covering the time between 7.30 am and 2.30 pm. Most hospitals work on a half-day basis during this period. The Government is expecting the new general hospital that is currently being constructed to operate on a full-day basis.

This would, however, entail a radical restructuring of the working hours of hundreds of staff members.

Although official figures are not available, probably more than 90% of public employees in the health sector are members of trade unions. About 80% of doctors are members of the Medical Association of Malta, while over 97% of eligible professionals were estimated to be members of the Malta Union of Midwives and Nurses, although this professional organization was only established in 1996. Most negotiations with regard to collective agreements are carried out at a central level, either within the Ministry of Health or within the Office of the Prime Minister. Agreements usually run for three years.

Health care facilities and equipment are generally of a high standard. Since 1995 most capital investment has gone into the construction of the new acute general hospital that will replace the present general hospital in 2007. According to a recent survey, patients are on the whole highly satisfied with public health services (*Sunday Times* 2003). Professionals have identified two areas where human resource policy has failed: the lack of effective management and the failure to create supportive environments for health care workers. One of the major problems experienced by health care workers is overcrowding of acute hospitals, because of the difficulties of transferring elderly patients with social care needs to long-term care facilities. Health care workers face particularly difficult conditions during the winter, when wards tend to be filled beyond capacity, with resulting high workloads and stress. There is also inadequate cooperation between different health care professions.

The rigid bureaucratic system within the public sector is a barrier to the improvement of working practices. Another main barrier to change is the financial situation of the country. The Government is not able to improve the financial packages of its employees and this could block necessary reforms.

Performance management

Quality assurance in health care as a distinct concept is still in its infancy in Malta and quality assurance measures have not yet been systematically introduced. However, physicians are encouraged to participate in quality assurance initiatives either individually or as a group through a scheme that provides a lump sum financial award. Clinical audit is also not yet regularly carried out consistently and is left to the individual clinician.

In certain areas of the hospital, accreditation schemes have been instituted. As part of an international accreditation system, a benchmarking initiative has been carried out, involving Malta's main hospital and several international hospitals. Malta has also recently hosted an international benchmarking conference. The benchmarking initiative has served as an impetus to examine internal processes. A review of all hospital policies and processes is currently being carried out with the aim of developing formal policies and protocols.

Performance appraisals are currently only carried out for senior management positions in the civil service. These positions are tied to a three-year contract and after this period civil servants need to reapply for their position. Health care professionals have never participated in the performance management programme that is in place for general civil servants. A performance management programme for doctors was briefly introduced several years ago but soon discarded. It was superseded by the scheme encouraging participation in quality assurance initiatives. The increasing professionalization of nursing has resulted in the development of nursing guidelines, protocols and standards.

An important challenge for the development of performance management in Malta is a certain tension between clinicians and management. However, there is increasing pressure to measure the performance of physicians in terms of resource utilization and efficiency, although clinical autonomy is likely to remain strong in the future. Another challenge for the development of performance management is that information systems are not yet sufficiently developed to have an impact on daily management or clinical practice. Much information is either collected manually or not at all.

In the two hospitals that have introduced budgets managed at ward or unit level, financial resources saved through efficiency gains can now be reinvested into the ward or unit. This has improved the performance of the respective managers. In general, however, all incentives for staff need the prior approval of government and trade unions. There is thus little scope for innovative measures at local level. The extensive private sector, staffed by doctors and nurses whose primary employment is in the public sector, also acts as a barrier to the implementation of performance management policies, as health care professionals are resistant to interference with clinical workloads.

Regulation

Health care professions are regulated through the statutory bodies established by the Health Care Professions Act of 2003, one of the main aims of which was to bring Maltese legislation into line with the EU *acquis* on mutual recognition of professional qualifications. Four statutory bodies regulate the health care professions: the Medical Council (comprising doctors and dentists), the Pharmacy Council (responsible for pharmacists and pharmacy technicians), the Council for Midwives and Nurses, and the Council for Professions

Complementary to Medicine. Unlike in the past, the statutory regulatory bodies have the same roles and responsibilities and the same degree of professional autonomy.

The primary role of these bodies is to maintain registers of health care professionals. They are additionally responsible for monitoring the education and training of health care professionals, in conjunction with the University of Malta and the specialist accreditation committees. The councils also have a role in establishing criteria for continuing medical education. Other main tasks of the councils are to establish professional guidelines and codes of ethics and to investigate cases of professional misconduct or negligence, including the proactive investigation of complaints. As in other European countries, actions by health professionals in Malta are coming under increasing scrutiny and litigation is becoming more common. The Government nominates lay people to the councils. Specialist accreditation committees will have the role of regulating the standards for postgraduate training and education. An area requiring more attention in the future will be to strengthen the cooperation between the different regulatory bodies.

In addition to the statutory bodies, health professionals are organized in professional associations on a voluntary basis. The Medical Association of Malta (representing doctors) and the Malta Union of Midwives and Nurses also play the role of trade unions. The Medical Association of Malta has acted as a coordinating body for the medical specialist associations that have emerged in recent years.

All health care professionals are accountable to their respective statutory regulatory bodies for their professional actions. Health professionals employed in the public sector are subject to the rules and regulations of the Public Service Management Code, covering the conditions of recruitment, employment and disciplinary mechanisms for civil servants. All promotions and calls for job applications are controlled by a central body, the Public Service Commission, in line with the Maltese constitution. Owing to present economic constraints, the Government has effectively frozen employment. However, filling of vacancies in the health sector has continued, albeit at a slower pace.

Conclusions

The case of Malta illustrates the difficulties that a small country with limited resources and an ambitious health care workforce is facing. Despite the lack of comprehensive reforms in the area of human resources in health, a number of best practices can be identified.

One concern is the adoption of many family-friendly measures, aimed to stem the outflow of female professionals. The case of the geriatric rehabilitation hospital, entirely staffed by returning nurses, shows the impact such measures can have on human resources. Another promising initiative is the management of budgets for the running of wards at the mental health hospital. It illustrated how health care professionals were willing to take a more active role in the management of health services. Finally, regular meetings between the Government and the trade unions have gone a long way towards building trust between the various parties. Their formalization at the national and local level would be an important step forward.

While Malta faces many of the issues encountered in developing human resources in health in other European countries, it exhibits some peculiar features, such as its geographical position and its history of turbulent industrial relations. In addition, the country faces the challenges of a thriving private sector staffed mainly by public sector employees and the emigration of newly graduated doctors to the United Kingdom and the United States. Many future improvements in the area of human resources in health hinge on delivering sustained financial benefits. In the present difficult economic situation, however, these changes will be hard to achieve.

REFERENCES

Azzopardi Muscat N (2002). The EU accession process: How EU membership will influence the Maltese medical profession. *Malta Medical Journal*, 14(1): 9–11.

Azzopardi Muscat N, Dixon A (1999). *Health care systems in transition: Malta.* Copenhagen, WHO Regional Office for Europe, on behalf of the European Observatory on Health Care Systems.

German L (1991). *Landmarks in medical unionism in Malta 1937–1987.* Malta, Media Centre Publications.

Melillo, T (2001). *Combining a medical career with raising a family – implications for Maltese female doctors and the health service* [thesis]. Valletta, University of Malta.

MoH (2003). *First National Health Interview Survey.* Valletta, Department of Health Information, Ministry of Health.

National Statistical Office (2004). *Labour Force Survey.* Valletta, National Statistical Office.

Sammut M (2003). *State primary health care – addressing medical man power needs* [dissertation]. Valletta, University of Malta.

Sunday Times (2003). 81% satisfied with health services. The Sunday Times Opinion Survey, *The Sunday Times*, 31 August 2003: No. 1298.

Chapter 6
Norway

Are-Harald Brenne[1]

Context

Norway's health care system is predominantly financed through general taxation and, to a lesser degree, through out-of-pocket payments. The private health sector remains small and very few citizens have private health insurance.

In 2001, the administration of the national health service was reorganized, combining the tasks of a greater number of smaller administrative bodies. The Ministry of Health and Social Affairs has assumed overall responsibility for the health sector and within it the Directorate for Health and Social Affairs is responsible for the practical organization and implementation of health programmes. The independent Board of Health has delegated responsibility for standards and quality, while the responsibilities of the Institute of Public Health relate to public health in general (Mjøen and Liseth 2003).

Following the Local Authority Health Care Act of 1984, local municipalities became responsible for all primary health care. In 2002, ownership of all public hospitals was transferred from the counties to the Ministry of Health. Five regional health enterprises have been established, responsible for ensuring the provision of health services in their respective geographical area. They are accountable to the Ministry of Health, which issues "Letters of Instruction". These regional enterprises own the 70–80 hospitals in the country that have been reorganized to form about 35 managerially largely autonomous health enterprises (Møller Pedersen 2002; MoH 2003).

[1] This chapter was instigated and funded by the Norwegian Directorate for Health and Social Affairs. Research was carried out by staff at the Programme for Health Economics in Bergen. Jan Erik Askildsen headed the project and Are-Harald Brenne drafted this chapter.

Table 6.1 *Health professionals 1990–2002 (full-time equivalent)*

		1990	1995	2000	2002
Hospitals	Physicians	4 576	5 402	7 073	7 291
	Nurses including midwives	15 614	18 457	22 343	23 451
Psychiatric institutions	Physicians	742	886	1 141	–
	Nurses including specialists	3 309	3 857	4 660	–
Primary health care	Physicians	3 067	3 463	3 809	4 150

Source: Statistics Norway (http://ssb.no).

Table 6.2 *Trends in numbers qualifying as health professionals, 1990–2002*

	1990	1996	1998	2000	2002
Physicians	310	490	494	606	590
Nurses	2 520	3 421	4 144	4 043	4 084
Dentists	105	114	113	121	113
Physiotherapists	185	306	305	317	303

Source: Third report from the first health personnel recruitment plan.
Note: Figures for 2002 are provisional.

The Government developed two subsequent plans for the recruitment of health personnel in 1998 and 2002 respectively. The plans have two main elements: to estimate the future supply of and demand for health personnel and adjust educational capacities accordingly, and to fund further education and competence building for existing health personnel, which it is hoped will increase job satisfaction and facilitate recruitment. The Directorate for Health and Social Affairs is charged with estimating future supply of and demand for health personnel, in conjunction with Statistics Norway. According to these projections, the most significant future challenge will be to recruit enough auxiliary nurses. Compared to most other European countries, Norway is sparsely populated and there are many small and remote communities, with significant implications for the geographical distribution of health personnel.

Workforce supply

The number of health professionals has increased since 1990 across professions and health sectors (see Table 6.1).

There has also been an increase in the numbers qualifying as health professionals (see Table 6.2).

Since the beginning of the 1990s, Statistics Norway has developed a framework designated HELSEMOD for estimating the future supply of and demand for health personnel.

Physicians

A 1983 government report projected that there would be a surplus of physicians in the future, unless the educational capacity for physicians was reduced (Willumsen 1983). By the late 1980s it became evident that these calculations, leading to reductions in the number of university places for medical students, were mistaken. In 1989, the shortage of physicians in rural Norway led to a law giving the Government the authority to allocate physicians to rural areas, although this was never implemented in practice (Buhaug 1997). Since 1990, the number of physicians being trained has gradually increased, with an impact on the job market since the end of the 1990s. According to the "medium scenario" of the 2002 HELSEMOD report, the demand for physicians will be met by 2010.

While about 67% of currently working physicians are males, close to 60% of Norwegian medical students studying at domestic and foreign institutions in 2003, were female. Historically, a large proportion of Norwegian physicians have received their education abroad (Bertelsen 1998). The number of Norwegian medical students abroad, supported by the State Fund for Educational Loans, increased from 579 in 1994 to 1934 in 2002. Currently the most popular countries are Hungary, Poland, Germany and Denmark. The Government has also secured a small number of student places at foreign universities, amounting to 45 in 2003.

According to Statistics Norway, 14 984 physicians were working in the health sector in 2002, equivalent to a ratio of 300 inhabitants per physician. When measured in full-time equivalents in 2001, 60% of physicians were working in hospitals, 34% in the municipal health service, and 6% in specialist practices.

According to data from the Norwegian Medical Association, the share of physicians from abroad increased from 2% in 1990 to 15.5% in 2003, most (45.6% in 2003) coming from other Nordic countries. The share of foreign physicians is higher in rural areas. In 1999, about one-quarter of physicians in two of the most rural counties, Sogn og Fjordane and Finnmark, had foreign citizenship, while in the small municipalities of northern Norway fewer than half were Norwegians.

Geographical imbalances in the supply of physicians

It has always been more difficult to recruit physicians to positions in rural areas, especially general practitioners and those working in less popular specialties, such as psychiatry and community medicine. An important policy tool for improving the supply of physicians in rural areas has been the control of demand elsewhere. Since 1999, all publicly financed physician positions have required a permit from the Ministry of Health.

Nevertheless, recruiting general practitioners to northern Norway has become increasingly difficult. In 1997, 28% of all positions in primary health care in the three most northern counties of Norway were vacant, with a vacancy rate of 37% in the small municipalities with a population of less than 4000. The insufficient coverage of health services is in part compensated by visiting personnel (often on expensive short-term contracts) and by physicians on internships (Kjekshus and Tjora 1998). Despite the recruitment problems faced by rural municipalities, however, the relative number of physicians is higher in rural areas, as there is an inevitable requirement for more physicians to cover a defined population in small municipalities simply because of the diseconomies of scale (Foss and Selstad 1997).

Two of the most important factors pushing physicians away from positions in rural areas are the workload from emergencies and the isolation from other physicians and medical expertise (Kjekshus and Tjora 1998; Grytten, Skau et al. 2000; Andersen, Forsdahl et al. 2001). Especially in the municipal health service, local recruitment measures have been mainly targeted at securing a stable situation rather than at avoiding an acute shortage of physicians (Kjekshus and Tjora 1998). All municipalities are required to provide their citizens with emergency physician services at all times. Publicly funded general practitioners are required to participate in this service. The payment from this work is an important source of income for physicians working in rural areas but the workload can become burdensome for the individual practitioner in small and remote municipalities.

The distance to the nearest hospital is often long, which may make it necessary for physicians to treat patients locally who would otherwise have been referred to hospital specialists. Since 1993 there has been a telemedicine department at the University Hospital in Tromsø to assist physicians working in remote rural areas. The Norwegian Centre for Telemedicine had about 110 employees in 2003. In 2002, it was designated as the World Health Organization's first collaborating centre for telemedicine. Another measure used in some municipalities to address the problem of professional isolation is to provide municipal health and care services in the same building. Some places cooperate with nearby hospitals and have visiting specialist physicians (Kjekshus and Tjora 1998).

Nurses and other health care workers

According to Statistics Norway, Norway had 64 150 nurses in 2002, equivalent to one nurse for every 71 people. Approximately 10% of nursing graduates in 2001 were men. 2.5% of nurses were from abroad and had fewer than five years' employment in the Norwegian system. Within the Norwegian health care system, health managers are often recruited from the clinical professions, in particular among physicians.

Following the Municipal Health Service Act of 1984, municipalities were required to offer physiotherapy services. The demand for physiotherapists grew faster than expected and by the early 1990s a shortage was recorded. In 1992, scholarships for students of physiotherapy studying abroad were reintroduced and the domestic educational capacity increased. Towards the end of the 1990s, the supply of physiotherapists increased and it is currently large enough to meet demand.

As already mentioned, auxiliary nurses, who, in contrast to some other European countries, continue to play a role in the Norwegian health system, are the groups for whom the expected gap between supply and demand is highest. According to the "medium scenario", the unmet demand will be 24 340 in 2020. An important reason for this is that, in 1994, many adults were excluded from the education system for auxiliary nurses. The recruitment plan for health personnel for the period 2003–2006 mainly focuses on education and competence development, while also discussing the recruitment of auxiliary nurses from abroad.

The educational capacity for dentists was increased by 8% during the 1990s. The 2002 HELSEMOD projections predicted a steadily growing undersupply of dentists. More than half of Norway's dentists are over 50. Since 2004 a new dentist education programme has been set up at the University of Tromsø. From 2002 onwards, Norwegian students studying dentistry abroad have been eligible to receive scholarships covering tuition fees. It is also planned that more dentists be recruited from abroad (Helsedepartementet 2003b).

Other workforce supply issues

In 1997, the Norwegian Labour Administration started a health personnel recruitment project to actively recruit health personnel from abroad. By 2002, 393 physicians and 1067 nurses had been recruited, mainly from Germany, Finland, Austria, Italy, France and Poland. In 2004 the project was terminated and the recruitment of foreign health personnel is currently being conducted within the framework of the European Employment Service (EURES), covering the European Economic Area and Switzerland.

Education and training

Physicians

Four universities in Norway admit students into medical education programmes, with student numbers ranging from 80 to 225 in 2001. The admission criteria are the same for all four medical faculties, although they have their own curricula and are not subject to detailed government regulation or standardization.

Since 2002 the medical faculties have admitted about 10% of all students into special research pathways. These students generally follow the normal curricula and spend additional time on research, extending their education from six to seven years.

After six years of basic medical education, there is an internship period of 18 months, consisting of six months on an internal medicine ward, six months on a surgical ward and six months in general practice. Internships are concentrated in rural areas. Physicians from many countries outside the European Union also need to complete the internship period in order to receive a Norwegian licence.

There are thirty basic specialties, and eight medical and five surgical sub-specialties. In general, the minimum period for specialty training is five years, although it takes on average nine years to complete. Since 1982, the Ministry of Health and Social Affairs has been responsible for regulating specialist education, since 1998 in consultation with the National Council for Specialist Education of Physicians and Physician Distribution. The authority to certify specialists has been delegated to the Norwegian Medical Association.

The medical faculties in university hospitals are the main providers of further education for physicians. The Norwegian Medical Association has several education funds that, based on individual applications, can cover travel expenses for course participants. An important element of further education for general practitioners is the creation of small peer groups with 3–12 participants. General practitioner specialists need to be re-certified in Norway five years after their initial certification, with participation in peer groups at least three times a year being a mandatory requirement (Johannesen 2002).

There are no tuition fees for public education in Norway. Higher education students, both at Norwegian universities and abroad, currently receive about NKr 80 000 (€10 110) in scholarships and loans per year. Norwegian students studying at foreign universities also receive a scholarship to cover travel expenses and, for studies in selected fields, funds for tuition fees up to NKr 50 000 (€6300).

By changing the eligibility criteria for receiving tuition scholarships, the Government can influence the number of students more quickly than by changing domestic educational capacities. This device was used in 1992 to increase the supply of physiotherapists and physicians. Since 2002 students of dentistry have been eligible for tuition fee scholarships.

Nurses

Twenty-seven colleges offer nursing education, 22 of which are university colleges, while the remaining five are located at health institutions. The minimum requirement for nursing education is secondary school education.

In 2000 the Competence Reform made it possible for people without formal degrees to be admitted into higher education based on their "real competence". The most important impact of this on the health sector has been to improve the recruitment of auxiliary nurses. Many previously employed as assistants have been certified as auxiliary nurses.

Basic nursing education lasts three years. Half of the time is devoted to practical work, of which between 32 and 42 weeks are spent in health institutions. Nursing science is established as an academic discipline, with master's degrees and PhDs. Further education programmes leading to nursing specialist degrees normally require some clinical experience and take one to two years to complete. It is common for students to receive their salaries while attending full-time further education programmes, in exchange for a commitment to continue working for their employer afterwards.

Nursing education is regulated by the Ministry of Education through the so-called framework plans, containing standards on curricula, teaching and assessment methods and practice periods. After taking over public university colleges from the counties in 1994, the central government presented a new framework plan in 2000.

Regional health enterprises are responsible for providing students of nursing, medicine and other health professions with practical placements. Some university colleges have had difficulties in finding enough practical placements for their students, owing to a lack of economic incentives for the health institutions. Although several working groups have suggested that regional health enterprises should receive earmarked funding for practical placements (Helsedepartementet 2003a; NOU 2003), the Ministry of Health planned in October 2003 to instruct regional health enterprises to offer practical placements for students through the "Letter of instruction" for 2004 (MoH 2003).

The Norwegian Nursing Association has created a clinical specialist programme for further education, leading to the certification of nurses as clinical specialists, which so far has not been recognized by the Ministry of Education. The programme offers courses for nurses in full-time employment, with and without specialist education.

According to the Norwegian Nursing Association, by October 2003 about 720 nurses had been certified as clinical specialists. At least one of the regional health enterprises has integrated the programme in their competence development strategy. There are also clinical specialist programmes for other health professions, including auxiliary nurses.

Health managers

With the hospital reform in 2002, there has been an increased focus on leadership training within public hospitals. In 2003, the Ministry of Health instructed the regional health enterprises to enrol people from higher management within each health enterprise in a two-year education programme organized by the Centre for Health Administration in Oslo.

Since 1986, the Centre for Health Administration has offered a full-time education programme targeted at health personnel with work experience. This has now developed into a one and a half year master's degree in health administration. Since 2002, the centre has offered bachelor's and master's degrees in health management and health economics. At the University of Bergen a further education programme in health economics targeting people working full-time in the health sector has been offered since 2000. Since 2002, it has also offered a similar programme in health management. The University of Tromsø has offered a bachelor's degree in health management since 2003.

Many health managers have also taken general management degrees. These have mostly been offered by private education institutions, in particular the Norwegian School of Management.

Auxiliary nurses

Auxiliary nurse education is organized by the counties within the higher education sector. Traditionally, mostly women older than 20 years have undergone auxiliary nurse education. With the reform of higher education of 1994, younger people were given preferential access to auxiliary nurse education, leading to recruitment problems (Høst and Michelsen 2003).

Working conditions

General practitioners

Since 2001 the general practitioner service has been funded according to a capitation system based on patient lists. With the patient list system, every individual is assigned to a general practitioner and, although this is not obligatory, 97–98% of the population now have a regular physician. The reform aims to provide more stable patient–doctor relationships and to improve the coordination between primary and specialist levels of care.

Since the introduction of the reform, only general practitioners with a municipal contract working within the patient list system have been eligible to receive fee-for-service refunds from the national insurance organization. General practitioners receive a basic fee for each patient they have on their list, currently about NKr 300 (€40). The capitation payments constitute about 30% of their income, while the rest is covered by fee-for-service payments and patient co-payments. Overall, the reform has increased the salary of general practitioners. Physicians without any government funding can freely charge their patients and the number of entirely privately financed general practitioners in cities has increased in recent years.

In many small and rural municipalities it has become common to employ physicians directly. Municipalities have to maintain an emergency physician service and need a minimum number of staff, potentially leaving physicians with a small number of patients. The physicians receive salary and overtime payments similar to other employees, and the municipality keeps the fee-for-service income and the patient payments.

Specialists in private practice

The working conditions for specialists in private practice have remained largely unchanged for the last 15 years. It is not uncommon for hospital physicians to work in private practice in addition to a full-time job at a hospital. Until 1998 they had the same reimbursement system as general practitioners, based on fee-for-service, patient co-payments and basic grants. Since they were part of the specialist health service, they had contracts with and received their grants from the county instead of the municipality. In 1998 eligibility to receive fee-for-service refunds from the National Insurance Administration was removed for specialists in private practice without a contract with a county, in order to improve the supply of physicians in rural areas. After the hospital reform of 2002, regional health enterprises assumed the responsibility for specialist health services and concluded contracts with specialists in private practices, who continued to receive their fee-for-service payments directly from the National Insurance Authority.

Physicians in hospitals

As the shortage of physicians increased in the 1990s, it became common for physicians working in hospitals to work in excess of the normal 37.5 hours per week. As compensation, in the second half of the 1990s they received large salary increases, mostly relating to overtime and night shifts. In conjunction with the hospital reform of 2002, the basic salary was increased and payments for extra activities reduced.

Since the hospital reform of 2002, local negotiations have become more important. Negotiations are first undertaken by larger organizations of unions on issues affecting all employees, such as pension funds or sickness insurance. Each union then negotiates issues affecting only their members, establishing minimum levels of payment for different services carried out by physicians. As a third step, local negotiations are being completed in the hospital sector at the level of health enterprises.

Nurses

Before the hospital reform of 2002, the Norwegian Nursing Association had separate tariff treaties with the central government, the Norwegian Association for Local and Regional Authorities and the municipality of Oslo, which at the time owned hospitals. In 2002, a single tariff was established for all hospitals, and salary levels increased substantially. The negotiations for nurses and other health professions are organized in a similar way to those for physicians. After a liberalization of the labour market in 2000 permitted the use of temporary employment agencies, the private sector job market for nurses has increased, as have salaries in the private sector.

The Norwegian Nursing Association has for many years claimed that there is a workforce reserve of nurses, consisting of part-time nurses and nurses working outside the health sector. Because of a heavy workload and underpayment, a large number of nurses and auxiliary nurses employed in the health sector, in particular women, work part time (Sørensen 2001; Askildsen, Holmås et al. 2003). Absence from work because of illness is much higher among nurses and auxiliary nurses than among physicians (Kommunenes sentralforbund 2002).

Performance management

Miscellaneous government initiatives

Given the organization of the Norwegian health care system, in which the municipalities are responsible for primary health care and social services and the responsibility for specialist health services rests with the regional health enterprises, the central government's role in performance management is limited to the establishment and enforcement of guidelines and quality management. The Board of Health is responsible for monitoring compliance with minimum standards in the health sector and for processing complaints by patients. The Directorate for Health and Social Affairs provides the central government's main policy mechanism for encouraging the development of higher quality services, by organizing the development of guidelines, quality indicators, research efforts and administration of medical databases.

Many databases containing information on specific treatments or institutions have been set up on the initiative of individuals, hospitals and universities. Thirty-five such medical databases were funded by the Directorate for Health and Social Affairs in 2002. In addition to these specialized databases, the Norwegian Patient Register, administered by SINTEF (The Foundation for Scientific and Industrial Research) under government supervision, collects patient data from hospitals, such as age, sex, duration of stay and diagnosis according to diagnosis-related groups (DRGs).

There have been scattered efforts at hospital and regional level to develop suitable indicators of the quality of health services since the first half of the 1990s. After the central government's takeover of hospitals and the reorganization of the central health administration, the development and use of quality indicators has been formalized by the Directorate for Health and Social Affairs. For 2003, nine variables were selected by the Ministry of Health to be used as quality indicators at the national level, providing information to the public about the performance of hospitals.

Since 1997 the Ministry of Health has financed the independent centre for Health Technology Assessment, which is administered by SINTEF. The Centre completes 10–20 assessments each year.

Until the end of the 1990s, there was no national policy on medical guidelines. There are several hundred medical guidelines in existence, many of which were developed by the pharmaceutical industry. The Directorate for Health and Social Affairs has started to establish a framework for the development of medical guidelines.

Activity-based financing

Before 1997 the counties, which at the time owned nearly all hospitals, were financed through grants from the state. In 1997 a financing system was introduced which based 30% of the counties' expected hospital budget on DRGs and 70% on grants (Kjerstad 2000). In 2003, 60% of the income of regional health enterprises was activity-based and linked to DRGs. The regional health enterprises generally use the same remuneration system for their health enterprises as the counties did, although exceptions exist, such as for psychiatric hospitals, which are usually financed through grants.

Since the introduction of activity-based financing in 1997, the reported activity, weighted by DRG, has grown rapidly, by an estimated 12% between 2000 and 2004. According to a Green Paper of 2003, quality does not seem to have been affected negatively (NOU 2003). The Ministry of Health and Social Affairs has initiated steps to make the coding system more transparent and easier to use, and to improve its monitoring.

About 50% of the costs related to the treatment of patients in outpatient care at hospitals are financed through a separate reimbursement system. In many cases private specialists provide similar services to the hospital outpatient clinics, but are financed through a fee-for-service system. The Government plans to develop a new diagnosis-oriented reimbursement scheme for both types of services (MoH 2003; NOU 2003).

The National Insurance Authority finances health services delivered by health professionals in private practice. Physicians are remunerated according to a system in which fees for services are established through negotiations between the Government and the Norwegian Medical Association. The local offices of the National Insurance Authority used to check in detail one monthly report per physician per year, mostly to prevent the excessive use of laboratory tests. With the introduction of a new computer-based system, their efforts will concentrate on cases giving reason for suspicion.

One of the goals of the capitation system was to strengthen the role of primary care physicians. Under the capitation system, the grant that general practitioners receive is based on the number of patients, creating an incentive to increase the number of registered patients, while reducing the workload per patient and increasing the referral rate to specialist health care (Iversen and Lurås 1998; Carlsen and Norheim 2003). General practitioners working full time generally have an upper limit of 1200–2500 patients (Iversen 2003).

Regulation

Regulation of the physician labour market

In Norway, there has been a long tradition of government regulation of the physician labour market, designed to recruit sufficient physicians to rural areas and to ensure an adequate supply of specialists. In 1979–1984 and 1988–1989 temporary laws were enacted to restrict the establishment of new physician positions in urban areas (Buhaug 1997). In the 1980s the Ministry of Health and Social Affairs, the Association for Local and Regional Authorities, the municipality of Oslo and the physicians' union concluded two treaties that obliged municipalities and hospitals to apply for a permit if they wanted to set up a physician position. By the mid-1990s, when there was a large undersupply of physicians, some institutions, especially hospitals in large cities, started to employ physicians without the necessary permits. In 1998 a law was passed which made it necessary to have a permit from the Ministry of Health and Social Affairs in order to employ a physician in a publicly financed position. The law also established the National Council for Physician Distribution and Specialist Structure.

General labour market regulations

Since the beginning of the 1990s, private companies have increasingly been permitted to act as intermediaries in the job market. In October 2001, 500 health professionals were employed by temporary employment agencies, 170 of whom were nurses.

Since 1954, there has been a common Nordic labour market. After 1975, the Norwegian immigration policy concerning workers from non-Nordic countries became very restrictive. In 1994, Norway joined the European Economic Area (EEA) agreement, subscribing to free movement of labour from EEA member countries. In 2000, the parliament relaxed the qualification requirements for immigrants. Since 2002, an annual quota of 5000 work immigrants has been set. When the quota is met, the qualifications of applicants are more closely examined. In 2002, 1676 people, mainly from eastern Europe and North America, were given work permits based on this regulation. Most immigrants, however, come as refugees or asylum seekers or through family reunion.

The Board of Health

The Board of Health, created through the reorganization of governmental health institutions, is mainly concerned with inspecting and controlling the health care sector. Its local offices supervise compliance with legal standards, regulations and internal control routines. The board also handles complaints from patients (Statens Helsetilsyn 2003).

The Registration Authority for Health Personnel

Licensing of health personnel has become an increasing concern in the last 15 years, in view of the increasing number of people with foreign education. Prior to the reorganization of governmental health organizations, the Registration Authority for Health Personnel was part of the Board of Health. Since 2002, it has been supervised by the Directorate for Health and Social Affairs. The Norwegian Medical Association and the Norwegian Dental Association certify specialists in their professions.

The Registration Authority for Health Personnel compares foreign with Norwegian education programmes. For health personnel from other Nordic countries there are no special requirements. Health personnel from the EEA are generally required to take courses or to document their proficiency in the Norwegian language and medical terminology. Applicants from the United States, Canada, Australia and New Zealand usually qualify directly and only have to take language tests.

For dentists and physicians, there are compulsory education programmes for those from countries outside the European Union. In order to gain authorization, physicians have to pass tests in Norwegian and Norwegian medical terms, pass a multiple-choice test, work for six months under supervision at a Norwegian hospital, complete a six-week training course, and complete an 18-month internship.

There are no mandatory educational requirements for nurses from countries outside the EU, except for a three-week training course. Applicants for authorization may have to complete specific modules of nursing education and some nursing schools offer customized courses for foreign nurses.

It is currently being discussed whether criminal records related to narcotics or sexual harassment offences should be considered when licensing health personnel. Another issue currently under discussion is whether the moral suitability of health personnel should be assessed during their education, in a manner similar to the regulations in place for teachers-to-be (Utdannings- og forskningsdepartementet 2003).

Conclusions

The Norwegian example illustrates the difficulties of planning the supply of health personnel. It also shows the importance of reacting quickly when estimates turn out to be wrong. Reliance on erroneous estimates had serious consequences for the Norwegian health care system throughout the 1990s. It is hoped that the establishment of a health personnel recruitment plan will enable the Government to act faster in the future.

The supply of physicians in rural areas has been a political problem in Norway as long as there have been physicians in public service. Professional isolation and the burden imposed by providing emergency care are important factors negatively influencing the recruitment of physicians. It is therefore very important for small communities to find ways to establish a stable physician workforce or to explore other ways of meeting their needs.

REFERENCES

Andersen F et al. (2001). Lack of doctors in rural districts – the situation in northern Norway, a national challenge. *Tidsskrift for den Norske Laegeforening*, 121(23): 2732–2735.

Askildsen JE et al. (2003). Wage policy in the health care sector: a panel data analysis of nurses labour supply. *Health Economics*, 12: 705–719.

Bertelsen T (1998). *De skapte legemangelen: Kampen mot utenlandsmedisinerne: En universitetspolitisk og profesjonspolitisk studie fra årene 1945–1960. [They created the physician shortage: the battle against physicians educated abroad. A study of university and profession policies in the years 1945–1960]*. Bergen, Alma Mater.

Buhaug H (1997). *Evaluering av Utvalg for Legestillinger og Stillingsstruktur (ULS). [Evaluation of the Committee for Physician Positions and Position Structure]*. Trondheim, Norsk Institutt for Sykehusforskning.

Carlsen B, Norheim OF (2003). Introduction of the patient-list system in general practice: changes in Norwegian physicians' perception of their gatekeeper role. *Scandinavian Journal of Primary Health Care*, 21(4): 209–213.

Foss O, Selstad T, eds. (1997). *Regional arbeidsdeling [Regional work division]*. Tano, Aschehoug.

Grytten J et al. (2000). Type of contract and location of general practitioners in Norway. *Tidsskrift for den Norske Laegeforening*, 120(26): 3134–3139.

Hagen T et al. (2003). *Behovsbasert finansiering av spesialisthelsetjenesten [Financing the specialist health service according to need]*. Oslo, Government Administration Services, Information Department (Norges Offentlige Utredninger 1).

Helsedepartementet [Ministry of Health] (2003a). *Praksisopplæring i spesialisthelsetjenesten. Arbeidsgrupperapport [Practical training in specialist health care. Work group report]*. Oslo, Ministry of Health.

Helsedepartementet [Ministry of Health] (2003b). *Rapport. Tannhelsetjenesten. Geografisk fordeling, hensiktsmessig oppgavefordeling og samarbeid mellom offentlig og privat sektor [Report. Dental health services. Geographical distribution, appropriate division of responsibilities and cooperation between public and private sector]*. Oslo, Ministry of Health.

Høst H, Michelsen S (2003). Who will nurse us in our old age? On the erosion of social and cultural preconditions for care education. In: Philipp G, Heikkinen A, Lindgren A, eds. *Social competences in vocational and continuing education*. Bern, Peter Lang Publishing Group.

Iversen T (2003). *The effect of patient shortage on general practitioners' future income and list of patients*. Oslo, Health Economic Research Programme at the University of Oslo (HERO).

Iversen T, Lurås H (1998). *The effect of capitation on GPs' referral decisions*. Oslo, Health Economic Research Programme at the University of Oslo (HERO).

Johannesen L (2002). Smågrupper i etterutdanningen i allmennmedisin [Supplementary training of general practitioners in small groups]. *Tidsskrift for den Norske Laegeforening*, 122: 2241–2242.

Kjekshus LE, Tjora AH (1998). *Hvor reell er mangelen på leger? En kartlegging av legebemanningen i et fylke [How real is the lack of physicians? A survey of the physician recruitment situation in one county]*. Trondheim, Norsk Institutt for Sykehusforskning.

Kjerstad E (2000). *Prospective funding of somatic hospitals in Norway: Incentives for higher production?* Bergen, Health Economics in Bergen (HEB).

Kommunenes sentralforbund (2002). *Kommunale arbeidstakere, fraværsstatistikk 2001–2002 [Municipal employees, statistics of absence 2001–2002]*. Oslo, Kommuneforlaget.

Mjøen G, Liseth S (2003). *Et direktorat blir til: hvordan kan vi ved hjelp av en normativ model foreta en empirisk analyse og forstå endringsprosessen som førte til opprettelsen av Sosial- og Helsedirektoratet [The creation of a directorate: how can we with the help of a normative model conduct an empirical analysis and understand the process of change that led to the establishment of the Norwegian Directorate for Health and Social Affairs]* [thesis]. Copenhagen, Nord-Trøndelag University College, Sør-Trøndelag University College and Copenhagen Business School.

MoH (2003). *Inntektssystem for spesialisthelsetjenesten [Remuneration system for the specialist health service]*. Oslo, Ministry of Health (White Paper No. 5 (2003–2004)).

Møller Pedersen K (2002). *Reforming decentralized integrated health care systems: theory and the case of the Norwegian reform*. Oslo, Health Economics Research programme at the University of Oslo (HERO).

NOU (2003). *Behovsbasert finansiering av spesialisthelsetjenesten [Financing the specialist health service according to need]*. Oslo, Statens forvaltningstjeneste. Helse departementet.

Sørensen BA (2001). *Et nytt helse-Norge? En panelstudie fra somatiske sykehus [A new health-Norway? A panel study from somatic hospitals]*. Oslo, Arbeidsforskningsinstituttet.

Statens Helsetilsyn (2003). *Tilsynsmelding 2002 [Annual supervision report 2002]*. Oslo, Statens Helsetilsyn.

Utdannings- og forskningsdepartementet (2003). *Høringsutkast til forskrift om skikkethetsvurdering i lærer-, helse- og sosialfagutdanninger i høgre utdanning [Proposal submitted for comments on regulation of security assessments of students in higher teacher and social- and health care education]*. Oslo, Ministry of Education and Research.

Willumsen E (1983). *Helsetjenesten i Norge [The Norwegian health service]*. Oslo, Health Directorate.

Chapter 7

Poland

Monika Strózik

Setting the context

Prior to 1989, health care in Poland was organized according to the Soviet Semashko model, in which the state was responsible for the financing, regulation and provision of health care. The post-communist health care system that has gradually evolved since the political transition is based on three principles: the redefinition of responsibilities for health care, the creation of a health insurance system, and the separation between payers and providers of health services. This has led to the emergence of new stakeholders in the health sector; local governments, for example, have assumed responsibility for aspects of health care, such as health promotion services, and have assumed ownership of almost all health facilities.

The health insurance system, membership of which is compulsory, began operating in January 1999. Individuals contribute 7.75% of their taxable income, with additional funds from government revenues for those who are unable to pay. The system was initially decentralized, with regional sickness funds established in each of the 16 regions (*voivodships*); which negotiated contracts with health care providers on behalf of their members. In January 2003, the regional sickness funds were amalgamated to create a National Health Fund.

The introduction of health insurance has changed the organization of health care provision. Sickness funds enter into contracts with health care providers who provide a defined package of services for the insured. The notion of choice plays a significant role. Patients can choose the health care provider, introducing an element of competition, with the financial resources of public and private health care providers coming from contractual agreements with health insurance funds.

Another element of health care reform in Poland has been the introduction of the concept of family medicine. This aims to strengthen primary care, with the general practitioner acting as a gatekeeper to more specialized care. Patients are allowed to choose freely among the general practitioners.

Workforce supply

In 1999, 14.6% of the total workforce in Poland was employed in the health sector (World Bank 2001). Available data on health care workers in Poland, however, are incomplete, as they do not take account of individual practices and may thus understate the supply of health care workers. In addition, employment categories have undergone several transformations in recent years, impeding a consistent classification of different professions. Based on data from public and private health care providers, but excluding single practices, there were 2.3 physicians and 4.9 nurses per 1000 population in 2001.

Compared to the 15 countries that were EU members prior to May 2004, Poland has a lower number of physicians and nurses per population. According to the WHO Regional Office for Europe Health for All database, in 2002 there were 2.3 physicians per 1000 population in Poland, compared to 3.6 in the 15 EU countries before May 2004. In the same year, there were 4.9 nurses per 1000 population in Poland, compared to 8.2 in the 15 EU countries before May 2004.

Over the course of the 1990s, the number of physicians per 1000 population has remained more or less constant. The number of nurses, however, has decreased from 5.4 per 1000 population in 1990 to 5.0 in 2002. There has been an even more pronounced decrease for dentists, from 0.5 per 1000 population in 1990 to 0.3 in 2001, while the number of pharmacists has increased (see Table 7.1).

There have been considerable regional differences in the distribution of health personnel. In 2001, there were 2.8 employed physicians per 1000 population in the region of Mazowieckie, compared to 1.4 in the region of Warmińsko-Mazurskie. 75% of health care staff work in urban areas, where only 65% of the population live.

Compared to countries belonging to the EU prior to May 2004, Poland has a high number of specialists, amounting in 2001 to 1.9 per 1000 population. There is in particular an oversupply of hospital doctors and specialists and an undersupply of physicians working in primary care, especially in rural areas.

Table 7.1 *Number of health care professionals in Poland per 1000 population*

Year	Physicians	Dentists	Nurses	Midwives	Pharmacists
1990	2.14	0.48	5.44	0.63	0.40
1995	2.32	0.46	5.48	0.63	0.50
1996	2.35	0.46	5.57	0.64	0.52
1997	2.36	0.46	5.62	0.64	0.53
1998	2.33	0.45	5.51	0.63	0.53
1999	2.26	0.34	5.10	0.59	0.52
2000	2.20	0.30	4.91	0.57	0.57
2001	2.24	0.26	4.82	0.57	0.62
2002	2.30	0.28	4.86	0.57	0.64

Source: WHO (2005).

As already mentioned, one of the aims of health sector reform has been to increase the emphasis on primary care. The share of employed physicians working in the primary care sector has increased from 16% in 1998 to 26% in 2001. However, the specialty of family medicine is still comparatively new. The first 300 family doctors completed training in 1994. In 2002, there were 5439 physicians possessing a specialization in family medicine.

The ratio of dentists to population in 2002 was 0.28 per 1000 population, about half of the average for the countries belonging to the EU prior to May 2004. There is a strong regional disparity in the distribution of dentists. The rate per 1000 population varied between 0.25 and 0.79 in the different regions of the country, with the highest density in urban areas and big cities.

The Polish Chamber of Physicians has received requests for physicians from several European countries. It has been estimated that since 1995 about 16 000 physicians have left Poland to work abroad (Michalak and Sieradzki 2003). In February 2001, the Norwegian and Polish National Labour Offices signed an agreement on the employment of Polish health care staff in Norway. Poland may face an increased brain drain in the years to come, although it may also experience an inflow of doctors from other EU Member States.

Throughout the 1990s, there has been a steady decrease in the number of dentists, although it is still considered to be too high. However, the available data are incomplete, as many dentists have opened private practices and their numbers are not captured adequately by regional health departments.

The Polish health care sector employs significantly more women than men. In 2001, women constituted 53.9% of physicians, 75.5% of dentists, 84.8% of pharmacists and 90.1% of laboratory assistants employed in the health sector.

There has been a growing role for public health specialists and health care managers in recent years, although they are still few in number. There is an insufficient number of positions for those who have undergone university training in public health and the positions available are not well remunerated. Health care units are generally run by physicians with no training in management or finance. Nurses still constitute a very small share of health care managers.

In 2002, there were about 190 000 economically active nurses, equivalent to 4.86 nurses per 1000 population. 15% of employed nurses were working in the primary care sector. As with physicians, there are regional differences. The number of nurses varies from 5.8 per 1000 population in the region of Lubelskie to 3.9 in the region of Wrmińsko-Mazurskie, the latter having the highest overall unemployment rate in Poland.

Fifteen thousand qualified nurses were unemployed in 2001, equivalent to 7.9% of the total number of employed nurses. Unemployment among nurses, however, is due to general economic problems rather than to an oversupply of nurses. As accommodation costs are very high in relation to the comparatively low salaries in the health sector, many nurses refrain from internal migration to urban areas, leading to unemployment of nurses in rural areas, while at the same time shortages of nurses occur in larger cities. Despite this low level of internal mobility, many nurses have expressed their willingness to work abroad. However, this would entail costs for language training and travel and many may work in less-qualified positions in the countries of destination. It can nevertheless be assumed that EU accession will facilitate the emigration of nurses, although the impact of accession is as yet unclear. The accessions of Spain and Portugal were only followed by very modest migratory movements (European Commission 2001). So far, Polish nurses trained in palliative care and operating theatre work have been recruited by Italy and Germany and there has also been recruitment of Polish nurses from Saudi Arabia, the Netherlands, the United Kingdom and the United States. At the same time, however, many professionals who have been working abroad returned to Poland in the 1990s.

As there will be an increasing demand for nursing services in the future, owing to the ageing of the Polish population, the country, like many others in Europe, is likely to face nursing shortages. The Government envisages an increase in the number of nurses and midwives employed to 345 000 by 2010, equivalent to an annual inflow of 10 000–17 000 nurses. To make the nursing profession more attractive for school leavers, it will be important to improve the professional and educational status of nurses.

Education and training

There are 11 medical academies in the country, constituting the main institutions for the training of health professionals in Poland. Within the higher education system, there are two different levels of education: a bachelor's level based on three years of study and a master's level based on five to six years of study.

Undergraduate medical training lasts six years (five years for dentists), followed by an obligatory internship. A national examination for medical students completing their internship was introduced in 2004. Passing the exam will be a major condition for obtaining the right to practise. In 1998, 14 751 students pursued medical studies and 2346 graduated. Admissions to medical faculties have been significantly restricted during the last decade. Until 1987, 6300 students per year were allowed to commence medical studies. This number was reduced in subsequent years and between 1994 and 2000 the annual intake was set at 2070 students.

Following their medical studies, students are required to undergo an internship, which lasts 13 months for physicians and 12 months for dentists. A new internship programme entered into force in 1999. Internships are now restricted to authorized health care providers and will be extended to psychiatry and family medicine.

Specialization after the internship takes three to seven years, depending on specialty. Preservative dentistry takes a minimum of three years, family medicine, public health and prosthetic dentistry a minimum of four years and other medical specialties a minimum of six years. During recent years, some new specialties have been introduced, such as family and emergency medicine. The training for the specialty of family medicine has been extended from three to four years. An alternative short course in family medicine now lasts one year instead of six months as previously. Emergency medicine was established as a specialty in 2000.

Although training schemes for dentists vary widely across EU Member States, the Polish system is very similar to the training provided in Germany or Belgium. EU directives require three years of practical training for dentists. Following the confirmation by the European Commission that Polish training programmes for dentistry comply with the *acquis communautaire*, the body of EU legislation, Poland changed the title of graduate dentists in 2001 from "doctor of dentistry" (*lekarz stomatolog*) to "dentist" (*lekarz dentysta*).

Between 1995 and 2000, dentistry faculties had an intake of 713–732 students per year. Although the number of students obtaining state funding was restricted, a larger number of students could study if they paid fees.

This practice has resulted in a large number of graduates, many of whom have difficulties finding employment.

The training of pharmacists was found to generally conform to EU regulations, with the exception of an earlier obligatory one-year internship following graduation, a requirement which has now been lifted. Pharmacy graduates receive a minimum of six months' training in a pharmacy during their studies and are able to practise independently upon graduation.

The specialist training is concluded with a national specialization exam, carried out by the Medical Examination Centre. This centre is accountable to the Ministry of Health and has responsibility for specialty examinations, continuing professional development, appointments to medical academies and the monitoring of curricula. Curricula and training programmes for specialties are prepared by groups of experts appointed by the Ministry of Health. The Ministry of Health also determines the number of places available for specialist training each year. Within their specialist training, physicians can compete for employment posts as residents. The financial resources for residency training are provided by the Ministry of Health.

Master's courses in public health are now available at several medical academies and other universities. Education of public health specialists started in 1994. Several private universities offer postgraduate courses in health management. The majority of graduates from postgraduate management courses are physicians, and many are hospital directors. Another large group of students work in health insurance funds or regional health departments.

Nurses used to be trained on a five-year vocational course that led on from secondary school. In 1991, nursing training was upgraded to a two and a half year vocational programme for candidates who had completed secondary education. The accession negotiations with the EU accelerated the reform of nursing education. EU directives required more hours of study for nurses than were provided for in the Polish education system. Nursing education now requires three years of higher education (resulting in a bachelor's degree), with a possible extension to five years (resulting in a master's degree). The amendment allows for the mutual recognition of the diplomas of nurses and midwives within the EU.

Nursing faculties have opened in five university schools of medicine and additional postgraduate training is now available in midwifery, paediatric nursing, psychiatric nursing and other specialties. Since the academic year 2001–2002, all medical academies and some higher vocational schools have been offering a bachelor's degree in nursing and midwifery. In the academic year 2003–2004, recruitment to vocational nursing schools ended. For graduates of nursing schools, a one year internship is now required for the right to practise the profession. The Accession Treaty of April 2003 ensured that qualifications of nurses and midwives with university education would automatically be recognized within the EU. Since the academic year 2003–2004, bridging courses have been provided for nurses or midwives who graduated from nursing schools. Although only 2% of all Polish nurses have so far obtained a university degree, the number of graduates is rising.

Postgraduate training of nurses has been based on modules undertaken during vocational education. Training courses are offered by authorized institutions for specialist qualifications in 26 fields of nursing or midwifery.

In 2001, the National Accreditation Council for Medical Education was set up. The Council accredits educational facilities for three to five years.

Working conditions

The structure and organization of health service provision is directly linked to the regional administration of the country. At the level of the commune (*gmina*), primary care services are provided. More specialized ambulatory care, including surgery, paediatrics, internal medicine and obstetrics/gynaecology, is provided at district (*powiat*) level. At regional level, highly specialized services are provided.

In the years after 1989, the public health sector faced a severe financing crisis. However, it did not collapse, as it was kept alive by formal and informal payments by patients. Households had to spend an increasing proportion of their disposable income on health care, while public health institutions accrued substantial debts. The health care reforms initiated at the end of the 1990s aimed to give the health care system a sustainable financial basis. Public health care institutions now compete with private providers for contracts with health insurance funds.

With the introduction of the health insurance system, competition between service providers has been encouraged. In 1990, physicians, dentists, psychologists, nurses and midwives were allowed to operate private practices. Privatization sought to improve the quality of health services, and to provide patients with easier access to physicians. One change in this direction has been the introduction of private practices of family doctors or dentists. When private providers sign contracts with health insurance funds, they are granted certain privileges associated with public providers, such as the licence to prescribe pharmaceuticals at reduced costs and free referral to hospitals.

In 1999, of a total of 791 hospitals, only 22 were private. In 1998, there were only 770 private practices, but it has been estimated that about 30% of doctors and more than 90% of physicians are involved in private practice (NERA 1997). In 1997, 45 000 physicians and 18 000 dentists were working in the private sector, compared to 91 000 physicians and 18 000 dentists in the public sector (Central Statistical Office 1998).

Health care workers in private institutions are generally more motivated than those working in the public sector. One study has shown that the number of consultations provided by dentists on fee-for-service contracts, for example, was more than double that provided by dentists employed in public health institutions (Chawla, Berman et al. 1998). There have been increasing numbers of nurses and midwives entering contracts with health insurance funds. In 1999, about 1000 contracts were signed with nurses and midwives. In 2000, this number had increased to 2431.

The mechanism through which providers are reimbursed by health insurance funds for their services has not been adequately regulated. Health insurance funds are free to decide the manner of payment. However, typically, specialists receive fee-for-service payments and acute care hospitals are paid for cases or a package of services, while long-term care institutions are paid per day of treatment. Virtually all payment schemes set a payment ceiling.

One of the forms of financing that has been widely accepted is the capitation method for primary care. The fee per patient is usually modified by the age structure of the population and other factors, such as the geographical distance to enrolled patients. Family physicians are also allocated funds for services provided by others, such as diagnostics or rehabilitation. While this was intended as an incentive for family physicians to treat patients themselves, instead of referring them to specialists or hospitals, there is currently no monitoring system in place that ensures that family physicians actually fulfil their gatekeeping role. There is also a lack of incentives to restrain prescription of tests or pharmaceuticals. Financing mechanisms similar to those for family physicians have been introduced for family nurses.

Unions and professional associations have played an important role in shaping the content of health reforms, in particular with regard to the payment of health professionals. After the implementation of health reforms in 1999, there have been a series of strikes and demonstrations. The protests were triggered by low salaries and the threat of unemployment. In 1999, the Government promised to increase salaries by 2% above inflation in all health care institutions. A further salary increase was envisaged by the Government in 2001. In the majority of health care units, however, a lack of financial resources meant that salary increases were not implemented.

The minimum level of pay is determined in a collective bargaining process involving trade unions or professional associations at the national level. At the workplace, negotiations take place between the employer and the trade organization that represents employees at local level. They are concerned with employment conditions, such as salaries and working times.

In 1974 a 40-hour working week was established for public employees in the health sector. This maximum working time was confirmed in 1991 and 2003. Implementation of the EU Working Time Directive, which limits working time to 48 hours per week, will nevertheless be difficult. A judgement of the European Court of Justice of September 2003 established that on-call duties count as regular working hours, which had not previously been the case in Poland. In addition, the limitation to 48 hours per week may force employers to increase the number of health personnel.

Until now, in the public health care system, all professional groups have been paid according to standardized employment contracts with fixed salaries. Remuneration was determined on the basis of qualifications and work experience and in comparison with other public salaries. In addition, health personnel received an annual bonus, the "thirteenth salary". Crucially, the salary thus did not depend on performance. Managers of public health care institutions negotiate their contracts directly with the regional health authority.

Pay levels, working conditions and morale remain problematic among health care personnel in Poland. As in other post-communist countries in central and eastern Europe, wages for health care workers were traditionally lower when compared to the workforce average. This has remained the case in Poland. Throughout the 1990s, the Government held down public sector wages in order to control inflation (Karski and Koronkiewicz 1999). In addition, all sectors of the economy faced a decline in real wages.

In 2002, the estimated average monthly salary in the health and social sectors was about €407, compared with an average monthly salary of €465 in the economy as a whole in 2003. There are important differences in the remuneration of different professions, although they are less pronounced than in many countries in western Europe. In 2000, a specialist with ten years' experience working in a city hospital received a monthly salary of €315. A nurse with the same experience working in the same workplace received €259. Salaries were considerably higher in the private sector. A nurse with ten years' work experience working in a private clinic in one of the major cities received €696 per month. In 2003, the average monthly salary for nurses was about €445.

Low salaries result in poor motivation and staff morale. As already mentioned, there is no incentive to work more than is absolutely necessary. Many physicians and dentists supplement their salaries in the public sector with private sector employment. In addition, as in the rest of central and eastern Europe low salaries are complemented by informal payments (Lewis 2000).

In Poland, informal payments range from small voluntary gifts to the extortion of large bribes (World Bank 1999). Although patients and doctors perceive informal payments rather as an expression of gratitude for the treatment provided, they may be considered a form of systemic corruption (Kubiak 2001). According to a survey conducted in 2001, the average informal payment by the patients participating in this survey was €139. The largest group in receipt of informal payments were directors of hospital departments and leading physicians. The professions with the lowest salaries (nurses and young doctors) tend to receive smaller informal payments or no such payments at all. The salaries of the majority of health care workers thus remain below the national average, even if informal payments are taken into consideration.

While young physicians without a specialization have difficulty finding employment, recorded unemployment among physicians is low. In 1999, only 0.6% of physicians were registered as unemployed.

Performance management

One of the most important activities for improving the quality of health services in the Polish health system has been the accreditation of health care providers. The institution tasked with the accreditation process is the National Centre for Quality Assessment in Health Care, which was set up in 1994 by the Ministry of Health. The main activities of the centre are:

- the accreditation of health care providers;
- the preparation of national guidelines and standards for medical procedures;
- the evaluation of medical technologies;
- the monitoring of quality indicators;
- the training of health care professionals.

By 2003, 59 hospitals had received accreditation. The accreditation certificates, which are valid for up to three years, are issued by the Accreditation Council on the basis of an evaluation conducted by the Centre for the Accreditation of Health Care Organizations. Although it is not yet obligatory, some health insurance funds take into account whether health care institutions have been accredited.

The accreditation requirements for hospitals include a section concerned with human resources management. One of the requirements in this area is the existence of a policy of continuing professional education. The accreditation of hospitals has significantly influenced the training of nurses and midwives, who have taken an active part in the accreditation process, according to a survey conducted in 2002 by the Council of Nurses and Midwives (Piskorz 2002). In all hospitals included in the survey, nursing was standardized and improved.

Accreditation for primary care does not yet exist. With regard to outpatient care and family physicians, the National Centre for Quality Assessment in Health Care, in cooperation with the College of Family Physicians, has created a draft version of accreditation standards. Prior to that, a voluntary accreditation programme was launched by the College of Family Physicians in 2001.

Regulation

Health professions are organized by statute into three associations, or chambers, membership of which is mandatory. The chambers cover physicians and dentists, nurses and midwives, and pharmacists. All oversee claims of professional malpractice and can revoke the permission to practise. District chambers represent each profession at regional level and maintain a register of eligible practitioners and private practices. The chambers also issue licences to physicians, nurses and midwives for private practice.

The main impetus for legislative reforms in the Polish health sector in recent years was the approximation of legislation to the *acquis communautaire*. In general, the legislation is prepared by the Ministry of Health, in consultation with professional bodies. The content of draft laws is then consulted upon with other relevant social actors, such as the trade unions.

In December 2001, Poland announced the (provisional) closure of negotiations concerning the chapter on the "free movement of persons". Following accession, EU citizens were awarded equal rights on the Polish labour market. Polish citizens will have equal rights in most other EU Member States after a transitional period, which ranges from two years (in Denmark, France, Greece, Ireland, Spain, the Netherlands and Sweden) to seven years (in Austria and Germany).

A key issue in the chapter on the "free movement of persons" was the mutual recognition of professional qualifications. In general, existing training programmes complied with EU regulations. An exception was, as already mentioned, the training of nurses. While EU diplomas and qualifications are now recognized in Poland using a fast-track procedure, the requirement that members of the medical profession must be able to speak Polish was maintained. Apart from this requirement, physicians from EU Member States have been given the right to provide services, become a member of professional bodies and establish private practices.

Conclusions

While there are still challenges ahead, the situation of health professionals in Poland has improved significantly during the last decade. In particular in the area of education, visible transformations have taken place. It will now be important to consolidate the new medical specialties that have emerged in recent years. Family medicine, which is situated at the centre of the health care reforms, needs particular strengthening. So far, there are an insufficient number of training posts, the duties required of family physicians are difficult to carry out and reimbursements provided by the National Health Fund are extremely low. It may be hoped that the implementation of accreditation procedures for family physicians will improve the efficiency and quality of services.

The upgrading of the education of nurses and midwives has improved their professional standing and enabled them to compete on the European labour market. Currently, however, only 2% of Polish nurses have completed university studies. It will be crucial to support nurses in pursuing bridging courses to upgrade their education and to facilitate continuing education. Training programmes will have to be financed at least partially from public sources. At a time of nursing shortages, with a decreasing number of candidates entering nursing education, EU accession might yet result in the emigration of young and well-qualified nurses. It would therefore be reasonable to train highly qualified nurses who could become trainers for less-qualified nurses. Such a move could be part of a more comprehensive effort to strengthen the professional role of nurses in the Polish health sector.

A final issue that merits attention is the working conditions of health professionals. At present, critically low salaries result in poor motivation, low-quality services, staff shortages and requests for informal payments. As long as resources in the health sector are restrained, avenues will need to be identified to address this situation.

REFERENCES

Central Statistical Office (1998). *Biuletyn statystyczny sluzby zdrowia [Statistical bulletin on health care]*. Warsaw, Central Statistical Office.

Chawla M et al. (1998). *Innovation in provider payment system in transitional economies: experience in Suwalki, Poland*. Boston, Harvard-Jagiellonian Consortium for Health.

European Commission (2001). *The free movement of workers in the context of enlargement* [information note]. Brussels, European Commission.

Karski JB, Koronkiewicz A (1999). *Health care systems in transition: Poland.* Copenhagen, WHO Regional Office for Europe, on behalf of the European Observatory on Health Care Systems.

Kubiak A (2001). *Pacjenci i lekarze o korupcji w publicznej sluzbie zdrowia – Raport z badan [Patients and doctors on corruption in public health. Research report].* Warsaw, Fundacja im Stefan Batorego, Program przeciw korupcji.

Lewis M (2000). *Who is paying for health care in Eastern Europe and Central Asia?* Washington, DC, World Bank.

Michalak J, Sieradzki S (2003). Biala emigracja [White immigration]. *Wprost,* 6 July 2003.

NERA (1997). *The health care system in Poland.* London, National Economic Research Associates.

Piskorz K (2002). Wplyw procesu akredytacji szpitala na funkcjonowanie obszaru opieki pielegniarskiej [Influencing accreditation processes in hospitals in nursing healthcare]. *Siódma Ogólnopolska Konferencja Jakosc w Opiece Zdrowotnej [Seventh Inter-Polish Conference on Quality in Healthcare, Krakow, 22–24 April 2002].*

WHO (2005). European Health for All database (HFA-DB) [online database], Copenhagen, WHO Regional Office for Europe.

World Bank (1999). *Corruption in Poland: review of priority areas and proposals for action.* Warsaw, World Bank.

World Bank (2001). *World Bank country study: Poland's labour market – the challenge of job creation.* Washington, DC, World Bank.

Chapter 8
Russian Federation

Kirill Danishevski

Setting the context

Since gaining independence following the dissolution of the Soviet Union in 1991, the Russian Federation has undergone a dramatic transition from communism to a market economy. A new constitution led to the devolution of power from federal to regional and local levels, while mandatory health insurance was introduced (Twigg 1999), spreading progressively to cover about 90% of the Russian population (Balabanova et al. 2003). So far, there is little private provision of health care or of voluntary health insurance, except in big cities such as Moscow and St Petersburg, although even there it is used by only a small elite.

The financing reform has not, however, been accompanied by a comparable change in health care delivery and the problematic legacy of the communist Semashko health care system persists, with an emphasis on curative and hospital care. Whereas official funding for health care remains relatively low, the number of hospitals in the Russian Federation continues to be much higher than the European average. Many aspects of the Russian health care system are ineffective, with high levels of avoidable deaths (Andreev et al. 2003); salaries of health professionals are low and informal payments widespread.

For most citizens of the Russian Federation, health care is obtained in facilities managed by their district (*rayon*) administration, to which the ownership of these state-run facilities was transferred in the early 1990s. These cover, on average, 15 000–50 000 people and receive about half of their funding from local budgets raised from general taxation. Typically, the central district hospital is responsible for administration of all facilities in the district. In addition, some larger, specialized facilities are accountable to the regional (*oblast*) health administrations (of which there are 89), with a few tertiary-level facilities owned by the federal Ministry of Health. These facilities receive part of their funding from regional or federal budgets respectively. Most health facilities also receive funding from the regional health insurance funds, which are accountable to regional governments and the federal health insurance fund (Chernichovsky and Potapchik 1997).

While the majority of health services are provided at the local level, the federal Ministry of Health and, to some extent, the federal Ministry of Education are responsible for higher medical education. This means that employers have very limited influence on the supply of health personnel, which is controlled and funded from the centre.

In the Soviet Union, graduates of general (non-paediatric or other) medical schools concentrated on a narrow area of specialization in their final year of studies. This system has been abolished, but graduates still tend to train for narrow specialties during postgraduate training. Most students receive financial support for their studies from the federal budget.

In addition to the mainstream Ministry of Health system described above, there are several parallel health services provided by various ministries (the largest being the railways, the military and the police), as well as by the more wealthy private and state-owned companies. Furthermore, even within the mainstream system, many specialties, such as obstetrics and gynaecology, paediatrics, general medicine and dentistry, work in separate outpatient and inpatient facilities in the larger cities. Sanitary-epidemiological (san-epid) services, responsible for surveillance, occupational health, environmental safety and the prevention of communicable diseases, form a separate vertical system, originally headed by a separate ministry, which was later integrated into the Ministry of Health but in 2004 again transformed into a separate institution as part of an administrative reform (President of the Russian Federation 2004).

In September 2003 the Russian Federation joined the Bologna Process, which seeks convergence of European higher education systems. It is intended that the Russian system will comply with European standards by 2010. Until then, foreign degrees are unlikely to be officially recognized in the Russian Federation. Currently, a diploma of higher education (awarded in most cases after five years of studies) is required for people wanting to work in the public sector. The private sector employs limited numbers of recently trained graduates with master's degrees. The existing licensing procedures mean that all physicians require a Russian diploma, even if they are working in private facilities.

Although there have been attempts to strengthen primary health care, reduce hospital capacity, and introduce modern public health and health management, most efforts have been in the framework of externally funded projects, with limited impact on the overall situation. The largest human resource reform initiative in the health sector, which sought to introduce modern general practice, with funding from the World Bank (Tver, Kaluga), the British Know-How Fund (Sverdlovsk, Samara, Kemerova), the United States Agency for International Development (USAID) (Saratov, Khabarovsk), the EU (Moscow area, Belgorod) and other international agencies, in conjunction with local initiatives, has produced only about 1500 GPs, representing less than 0.2% of all physicians in the Russian Federation (Rese et al. 2005). Meanwhile the Soviet version of a GP, the *Uchastkovii terapevt* (UT), physicians with a narrow clinical repertoire who serve as a primary contact for a geographically defined population and usually act as a referral point to secondary care, is dying out, as no new physicians are entering the profession.

Workforce supply

The health sector in the Russian Federation, including medical care, social care, and rehabilitation facilities, employs 7% of the working age population, totalling 4.5 million people in 2000. According to Goskomstat, the National Committee on Statistics, medical facilities employed 3 563 000 people, rehabilitation facilities 300 000 and social care 372 000 (Goskomstat 2001). Ministry of Health data, which are used in WHO databases, differ slightly, as they only cover the Ministry of Health system, whereas Goskomstat also collects data from parallel systems. There are also some minor discrepancies relating to the inclusion of various specialties, as pharmacists for example are counted as physicians by the Ministry of Health, but not by Goskomstat (MoH 2003c).

Physicians

The number of physicians in the Russian Federation increased to 680 000 in the late 1990s, reaching a ratio of 4.71 per 1000 population. 154 000 were specialists in internal medicine, 89 000 surgeons, 69 500 paediatricians, 55 000 dentists and 41 000 obstetricians and gynaecologists. 27 500 physicians were working in the san-epid system, while the remainder were working in other specialties, such as ophthalmology or otolaryngology. As already mentioned, only 1500 physicians have been trained in modern family medicine or general practice. It is not clear however, how many were actually working as generalists, as their place in the system remains undefined. Less than 4% of health care professionals are working in the private sector, mostly in the pharmaceutical industry. Two-thirds of physicians are female, although there is a marked hierarchical gender stratification; males are concentrated in the higher profile areas such as surgery and other specialties that attract higher incomes, such as urology or gynaecology, while females predominate in the first-level district facilities (MoH 2002).

Primary health care in general is greatly understaffed. Although official statistics have not been published by Goskomstat, it has been estimated by the Ministry of Health that about 120 000 salaried positions exist (MoH 2003a). In many areas, less than 50% of these positions are filled, with about half being staffed by pensioners.

Some authors claim that about 80% of physicians are employed in the hospital sector, although the European Health for All database provides an estimate of 46% (WHO 2003). The difference is probably due to whether dentists, san-epid specialists and specialists providing both outpatient and inpatient services are included in the denominator. According to the Ministry of Health, the number of inpatient positions in the Ministry of Health system in 2002 amounted to 513 618, compared to 204 888 outpatient positions (MoH 2003c). Most outpatient physicians have very narrow and limited specialist training. In addition, informal enquiries failed to identify a single physician graduating in Moscow who became a primary health care doctor (UT) in the 2000–2005 period. Regional reports corroborate this pessimistic picture: in the Tula region less than 7% of all physicians work as primary health care doctors, occupying half of the available staff positions. Smaller facilities that have two to three UT positions often seem better staffed than larger ones, where better alternative job opportunities exist (Regional Health Authority 2003).

While population growth in the 1990s was negative, the number of physicians increased from 667 300 in 1990 to 682 500 in 2000, resulting in an increase from 4.5 physicians per 1000 population in 1990 to 4.7 in 2000 (Goskomstat 2001). According to Ministry of Health data, the ratio was slightly lower, but, at 4.2 per 1000, still significantly higher than the European average of 3.6 per 1000 population (WHO 2003).

Nurses

The number of nurses decreased in the 1990s from 1 844 000 to 1 611 700, corresponding to a decline from 12.5 to 11.1 per 1000 population. 65% were general nurses, 10% midwives, 10% feldshers (nurse practitioners working in rural areas where there are no physicians) and less than 5% were specialized in laboratory diagnostics, radiography or dentistry. The Ministry of Health has estimated that over 99% of nurses in the Russian Federation are women.

The distribution of nurses by levels of care is skewed heavily towards inpatient services, where 74.4% of all nursing positions in the Ministry of Health system are located. Nurses are relatively well distributed among regions, although there might be disparities between rural and urban areas within regions. A shortage of nurses in bigger cities has led to an influx from neighbouring areas.

Health managers

The Russian health system is run by physicians. The heads of regional health administrations and of major federal and regional health management and financing organizations (such as health insurance funds) are almost exclusively physicians. In most cases they continue to work part-time as clinicians. Since the 1970s, district hospitals have taken over the role of local health administrations, making the head of the hospital responsible for the district health care system. Many clinicians have part-time administrative roles, such as deputy head physicians and heads of departments, which makes it hard to estimate the ratio of health managers to staff.

Although there have been attempts to develop health management education, so far only one regular health management programme exists, comprising two years of full-time training (*ordinatura*) in health management and public health. Outside medical education institutions, however, several programmes for health managers have been initiated, mainly training staff to work in the private sector. Most new graduates are not attracted by working conditions in the governmental health care sector, as they cannot compete for influential positions, which are traditionally occupied by senior physicians.

Nurses with sufficient work experience can be promoted to the position of senior departmental nurse. Despite the introduction of higher education in nursing, new graduates are generally unable to compete for senior positions and financial or status rewards are lacking.

Other categories of staff

Other human resource groups include specialists in "sanitary hygiene", recently renamed "preventive medicine". Preventive medicine departments are separate from medical departments and provide a graduate-level course lasting five and a half years, designed to train staff for the san-epid service. The specialty often attracts those who failed entry exams for other medical specialties. Although the san-epid service is based on an obsolete Soviet model, it has been maintained, partly because it is to a considerable extent financially self-sustainable. Part of its budget comes from fees charged to and penalties imposed on small businesses, creating many opportunities for corruption.

Social hygiene departments in medical academies, recently redesignated as departments of public health and health care, teach medical students, but also offer postgraduate specialty training in public health and health management. However, there are no obvious career opportunities within the health sector for specialists with this type of postgraduate training.

Medical assistants, *sanitars*, are in charge of transporting patients and cleaning and disinfection. This is an especially undersupplied group of personnel and most positions are occupied by medical or nursing students or by pensioners.

Workforce challenges

Two major problems relating to workforce supply are the imbalance between specialized hospital physicians and generalists working in primary health care, and the low ratio of nurses to physicians. The shortage of nurses and primary health care doctors seems to be at crisis level. Physicians are carrying out work that in western countries is done by nurses and generalists, while nurses are doing cleaning and other unskilled work, owing to the shortage of medical assistants. Another problem is the lack of a public health profession. Prevention, especially of noncommunicable diseases, is almost non-existent.

Despite comparatively low salaries, the number of physicians has been increasing. While in 2000, salaries of physicians were at only 80% of the national average, 95% of all positions were occupied (Goskomstat 2001), although most physicians occupy more than one position. Informal payments by patients are, however, believed to contribute to the constant supply of physicians.

Although the need to attract physicians to primary health care and to change the skill mix in favour of generalists has been proclaimed at all levels of health administration, it has not received the necessary support of senior health managers and the system has been ill-equipped to accommodate this change. As a result of the activities of western organizations, this issue has received more attention than others, such as informal payments or the shortage of nurses, but results are still unsatisfactory.

Education and training

The training of physicians in the Russian Federation is a centralized process predominantly coordinated and funded by the Russian Ministry of Health. The major exceptions to this rule are those universities which have a department of medicine, such as the Moscow State University, the International University of People's Friendship in Moscow, the Classic State University of St Petersburg and a number of smaller universities in Petrozavodsk, Ulianovsk and some other cities.

Postgraduate training and the retraining of medical specialists is carried out in educational institutions subordinated to the Ministry of Health. There are 47 educational institutions for training in the following specialties: medicine, paediatrics, dentistry, preventive medicine, pharmaceuticals, biological chemistry, and biophysics. They include 10 faculties of higher nursing education and 11 centres for general practice/family physician training. Continuing education for physicians is provided by 51 faculties in medical and pharmaceutical educational institutions. In addition, there are seven establishments of post-graduate medical education, in Moscow, St Petersburg, Irkutsk, Kazan, Novokuznetsk, Penza and Chelyabinsk. The majority of establishments for nursing education, 430 of 451, are subordinated to regional health authorities.

All curricula as well as major regulations concerning medical education have to be approved jointly by the Ministry of Health and the Ministry of Education. Despite some attempts to establish private medical schools in the mid-1990s, all have failed. The Department of Educational Medical Establishments and Human Resource Policy at the Ministry of Health is in charge of most training issues. It has several basic aims:

• organizational support of higher medical training;

• organization of postgraduate and additional training;

• development and approval of educational standards and curricula;

• certification, attestation and continuing development of medical staff.

The department, together with the Russian Ministry of Education, affirms the state educational standards and programmes, which include federal and regional components. It also develops the requirements for specialties for doctors, medical staff and pharmacists. Currently, 123 specialties are recognized, which is significantly more than in western Europe.

The educational requirements for physicians are ten to eleven years of school education, six years of medical education for medicine or for paediatrics, five and a half for preventive medicine and dentistry and five for pharmacists. Entrance examinations usually consist of Russian language, chemistry, biology and physics. Three to fifteen people compete for each place in medical training. Anecdotal evidence suggests that personal connections and bribery used to play a role in the selection process, although control has been tightened in recent years. Students from rural areas or men who have completed military service are given preferential access. Men who pursue medical education are exempted from compulsory military service, providing an additional incentive to enter the profession. After graduation, physicians generally follow one year of internship (*internatura*) or two years of residency (*ordinatura*) in their respective clinical field. All physicians are required to undergo one month of continuing education followed by an exam every five years, establishing their occupational category and salary level. Those who want to pursue an academic or management career path follow three years of *aspirantura*, a research degree similar to a western PhD, leading to the degree "Candidate of Science". This can be followed by three to four years of additional studies, leading to the submission of a thesis for the degree of "Doctor of Science". Practising clinicians receive higher salaries than academics, with the gap being widened further by informal payments, so that few qualified specialists are attracted by purely teaching and research positions. It is also worth noting that many physicians and about 50% of nurses do not obtain employment in the health sector after receiving their degrees (MoH 2003b).

The nursing profession can be entered after eight to nine or ten to eleven years of school education, followed by up to three years of nursing education, leading in both cases to a diploma in general nursing. This can be, but rarely is, followed by different programmes of additional specialization with or without interruption from work.

The number of students admitted to higher medical education institutions dropped from 24 800 in 1990 to 24 700 in 1995 but then increased again to 35 000 in 2000. The number of places in facilities for nursing education decreased from 114 000 in 1990 to fewer than 83 000 in 2000. 63% of physicians currently employed have undergone postgraduate specialization, but only 50% have taken part in continuing medical education.

Russian medical education has been influenced by international knowledge and research to only a very limited extent. A lack of language skills, poor access to the Internet, and limited library resources mean that few Russian academics have access to international medical literature. Their training was generally based on the Soviet model of science, with its emphasis on experts and experience, with a rejection of the concept of evidence-based medicine (Krementosov 1997). Currently, training during the first three years takes the form of lectures or seminars and modern teaching methods are mostly absent. In the final three years training usually takes place in hospitals, with complementary lectures and seminars.

Medical education continues to be confined to the narrow training of specialists. Separate undergraduate departments train physicians and paediatricians, complicating the introduction of family medicine. However, some changes were recently introduced concerning the final (sixth) year of medical studies. Until then, students of general medicine had to select one of the following fields of primary specialization: internal medicine, surgery, or obstetrics and gynaecology. In 2000–2001 this was changed, making it compulsory for all students to receive training in general practice/family medicine in the final year of studies. However, the continued existence of independent paediatric medical schools poses a barrier to the education of generalists or outpatient-oriented physicians in the Russian Federation. Some regions, such as Omsk and several others in Siberia, have responded by training child and adult GPs separately for the two existing systems of outpatient services.

Working conditions

According to the Ministry of Health, 95% of all active physicians in the Russian Federation work in the Ministry of Health system and most of the remaining 5% are employed in the parallel systems belonging to various ministries and industries. Salaries in the Ministry of Health system are paid according to the number of posts occupied (ranging from 0.25 to 1.5 staff positions), seniority, and the level achieved in continuing medical education. One of the major opportunities to supplement official incomes for physicians is by working 24-hour shifts; most do this up to six times per month. With a national poverty threshold of 1200 roubles per month in 2000 (about US$ 40), surgeons and physicians working in ambulatory care received 2400 roubles, remaining physicians between 1200 and 2400 roubles, and all nurses were below the poverty threshold. However, informal payments, in particular to physicians, complement official salaries and popular surgeons in Moscow were reported to charge US$ 1000–15 000 per procedure. Physicians who hold positions as health managers also receive higher salaries. Hospital managers receive extra benefits according to the number of hospital beds they are responsible for.

Until 2003, salaries were defined by a unified salary scale regulating all salaries in the public sector. There are still no negotiation mechanisms for the remuneration of physicians and they are not represented by a single professional association.

The long-standing tradition of Soviet-style control persists and any decision relating to salaries can be challenged by the tax department or various auditing and inspecting commissions. Head physicians who could provide additional benefits and premiums to their staff tend not to do so, as they risk penalties from inspectors, there are only limited incentives to recruit and retain better staff, and physicians seldom leave their jobs. However, arrangements are often made to raise the incomes of nurses, since they are in short supply and have few opportunities to receive informal payments.

Most conditions of employment are defined for the whole public sector. They provide for 24 to 36 days of paid holiday per year, up to three years of maternity leave, and a maximum working time of 40 hours per week (although as noted, most physicians supplement their income with additional shifts). A distinguishing feature of the Russian health care system is that in reality physicians have short working days, starting at eight or nine in the morning and finishing usually before three in the afternoon, constituting on average less than six hours. In outpatient care, physicians work either morning or evening shifts of five and a half hours. This enables them to work in more than one place or to occupy more than one staff position.

The workload per staff position is defined by official norms of the Ministry of Health, some of which have not changed since the Soviet period. For instance, a primary health care doctor serves a population of 1700 people and a paediatrician of primary contact (*uchstkovii pediatr*) serves 1200 children.

With regard to working conditions, facilities are generally not well maintained and equipment tends to be seriously outdated. Outside Moscow and those regions with large international projects, few physicians have access to computers (MoH 2003b).

There are strict hierarchical relations. Nurses are subordinate to physicians and have very little professional autonomy, while the hierarchy among physicians is even stricter and decisions of heads of departments are hardly ever challenged.

The working conditions of physicians differ in private clinics, as well as in state hospitals working with voluntary medical insurance companies, compared to others. The salary of physicians in the private sector in Moscow varies between 15 000 and 40 000 roubles (US$ 500–1200), while senior specialists can receive twice as much. Working hours tend to be longer, although they vary from clinic to clinic. In other matters, however, private clinics have copied existing models from public health care and the care provided is similar.

A policy successfully promoted in some places, including Yekaterinburg, Moscow and St Petersburg, is that of contracting. Instead of fixed staff positions, flexible contracts are used for nurses, physicians and managers, making it possible to increase salaries and responsibilities. However, contracted staff can only be paid after all budget lines have been funded and contracting arrangements are often challenged by tax departments.

Malpractice litigation or complaints are only possible against the institution concerned, but not against individual physicians. Only litigation where a criminal offence is believed to have taken place, such as one leading to death or severe injuries, can be instituted against an individual health care worker. As the system for complaints is complicated and as complaints are rarely taken to court, physicians are in effect unaccountable. There are about 20 organizations dealing with complaints, which makes it almost impossible for patients to claim their rights, as they are referred from one institution to the next. In addition, all of these organizations are run by physicians. Courts in most cases refuse to accept cases against medical workers, without giving further explanations (Russian League of Patient Defenders 2003). Complaints are therefore viewed by most patients as useless.

Performance management

Quality of care is a widely discussed but poorly institutionalized concept in the Russian Federation. Evidence-based medicine is one of the terms which has penetrated all layers of the medical community but remains poorly understood. In reality, user-mediated mechanisms for quality assurance in the Russian Federation are quite limited, owing to the traditional respect for physicians, and patients' lack of knowledge about their rights and sources of health information. Health facilities often retain a monopoly position, except in some large cities where federal, regional, municipal, parallel and private facilities create some degree of competition.

The main policies promoted by the Russian Ministry of Health with regard to quality assurance are continuing medical education and attestation and the promulgation of treatment guidelines. The system of continuing medical education, described above, does not include all physicians and treatment guidelines are produced in such a format that they are more suitable to define a package of services than to guide clinical practice. The Federal Laboratory for Standardization of Medical Practices was established in the late 1990s, but the first guidelines it developed were not user-friendly, were poorly distributed, and have rarely been used in everyday practice (Regional health authority 2003).

In medical education, research methods are very rarely and only briefly taught and there are very few peer-reviewed journals, allowing the pharmaceutical industry to relentlessly promote its products. Licensing procedures used for equipment, pharmaceuticals and facilities are aimed at quality assurance, but concentrate on safety, rather than on effectiveness or quality of care. In particular the licensing of pharmaceuticals is based on very small studies, often non-randomized and without control groups. The licensing of facilities is based on compliance with san-epid defined norms, fire safety and ensuring that all physicians possess diplomas.

The unfamiliarity with research methods makes evaluation of performance difficult. There is some anecdotal evidence, for instance, that statistical departments in municipalities manipulate infant mortality data to conceal chance variations, in order to avoid conflicts with higher level authorities.

The main method of guiding practice derives from the very strong hierarchy of health care in the Russian Federation. The heads of departments determine the methods used within their department and practices tend to be based on the knowledge and experience of senior physicians. The scope for quality assurance by professional associations is constrained by the early stage of development of these associations in the Russian Federation and the lack of qualified personnel independent from the state system. Although salaries usually do not produce perverse incentives, informal payments in many situations may do, leading to over-medicalization and supplier-induced demand.

Regulation

An important characteristic of the regulatory framework of the Russian health care system is the decentralization of responsibility and management to lower level health care organizations, while a strong hierarchy within organizations is maintained, backed up by strict financial regulations and inspections. Even though the great majority of regulatory documents produced by the Ministry of Health provide only recommendations, most health managers prefer to follow these regulations to the letter to justify their decisions.

There are two main groups of regulatory documents at federal, regional and local level: documents emanating from the legislature (laws) and documents emanating from the executive (orders or decrees and recommendations). Compliance with a decree from the Ministry of Health is obligatory if it has been approved by the Ministry of Justice. Although there is a special committee that deals with the development and approval of laws on health and sport, its work does not usually concern issues of human resources. The laws concerning human resources in the public sector tend to be not specific to health care and are often developed by other ministries and interest groups, such as the ministries of labour, taxation or railways, or lobbied for by large industries, such as mining. Most human resources issues, including working time, vacations, conditions of discharge and pension age, are defined by the Federal Law on Labour. However, there are several decrees and laws developed by the Ministry of Health which concern human resources issues, covering, for example, health insurance and the regulation of private practice.

While the Federal Law on Tariff Value regulates public salaries, additional payments can be made at the discretion of the management, for example based on profits from directly paid services or voluntary medical insurance schemes. The situation is complicated further by the fact that most health care is partially funded through the compulsory health insurance scheme, which is not an official part of the state budget. Although the salaries of most doctors are paid by the insurance scheme, the payment goes first to the budgetary facility, tying salaries of medical staff to budgetary law and the unified salary scale.

Other regulatory documents relevant to human resources in the health sector are those on licensing, with a number of decrees and orders of the Ministry of Health regulating the requirements for physicians and nurses of different specialties. A policy by the Ministry of Health which required that all doctors specialize in addition to their diploma was banned in the late 1990s, as it was found to conflict with the constitution. Instead, the Ministry of Health established a two-year residential training course and the re-certification of physicians every five years, but as mentioned above, not all physicians attend these training schemes. Finally, the criminal and civil codes regulate litigation in malpractice and other illegal cases, such as the inappropriate use of narcotics.

Initiatives to include professional associations in the processes of attestation and performance management are hampered by the early stage of development of professional associations. There are many weak and duplicating associations which lack democratic mechanisms of management and cannot sustain themselves financially.

Although the administration of health facilities does not usually allow for one person to occupy more than one and a half staff positions, the lack of physicians in primary health care has led to some younger physicians taking on three to four times as many patients as envisaged, with corresponding financial rewards.

Conclusions

Both the transition to a market economy and the introduction of a health insurance system have left the Semashko system of health care delivery almost unchanged. There continues to be an excess of hospital facilities and physicians compared to western countries. Low health care funding leads to informal charges as alternative sources of income are unavailable, a situation similar to that in other state sectors in the Russian Federation, including education, the social sector and the military. Primary health care and nursing jobs are unattractive for young graduates and remain understaffed. The lack of public health education, the dominant role of clinicians in health management and policy and the unclear division of responsibilities between authorities make quick and effective reforms in the near future unlikely.

However, there are also some positive developments. The signing of the Bologna Declaration, initiatives to introduce general practice and a public health profession, administrative reforms seeking to separate and to strengthen policy-making and control functions and the recent attention to health and demographic issues at the highest political level give rise to hope for an accelerated pace of reforms.

REFERENCES

Andreev EM et al. (2003). The evolving pattern of avoidable mortality in Russia. *International Journal of Epidemiology*, 32: 437–446.

Balabanova D, Falkingham J, McKee M (2003). Winners and losers: the expansion of insurance coverage in Russia in the 1990s. *American Journal of Public Health*, 93: 2124–2130.

Chernichovsky D, Potapchik E (1997). Health system reform under the Russian health insurance legislation. *International Journal for Health Planning and Management*, 12: 279–295.

Goskomstat (2001). *Zdravoohranenie v Rossii*. Moscow, National Committee on Statistics.

Krementosov NL (1997). *Stalinist science*. Princeton, NJ, Princeton University Press.

MoH (2002). *Health and health care in Russia: annual report*. Moscow, Ministry of Health of the Russian Federation.

MoH (2003a). Internal documents. Moscow, Department of Human Resources and Education, Ministry of Health of the Russian Federation.

MoH (2003b). Private communication. Moscow, Ministry of Health of the Russian Federation.

MoH (2003c). Private communication and internal documents. Moscow, Department of Statistics, Ministry of Health of the Russian Federation.

President of the Russian Federation (2004). *Decree on system and structure of federal organs of executive government No. 314 of 9 March 2004*. Moscow, Russian Federation.

Regional Health Authority (2003). Private communication. Regional Health Authority of Tula and Tver.

Rese A et al. (2005). Implementing general practice in Russia: getting beyond the first steps. *BMJ*, 331: 204–207.

Russian League of Patient Defenders (2003). Private communication.

Twigg J (1999). Obligatory medical insurance in Russia: the participants' perspective. *Social Science and Medicine*, 49: 371–382.

WHO (2003). European Health for All database (HFA-DB) [online database]. Copenhagen, WHO Regional Office for Europe.

Chapter 9
Spain

Beatriz González López-Valcárcel, Carmen Delia Dávila Quintana,
Elena Rodríguez Socorro

Context

The Spanish health care system is an integrated national health service that is publicly financed from general taxation and provides nearly universal health care free of charge at the point of use (Rico 2000). Provision is mostly in publicly owned and managed facilities.

Spain comprises 17 regions (the autonomous communities), with those on mainland Spain having between 7.2 million (Andalucia) and 264 000 inhabitants (La Rioja). The most significant institutional reform implemented in recent years was a process of decentralization, devolving responsibility for health care from the national health system to 17 regional health services in January 2002. Until then, only 7 of the 17 regions had this level of autonomy. Before this change took place, INSALUD (*Instituto Nacional de la Salud,* or National Health Institute) was responsible for publicly funded health care in the 10 non-autonomous regions.

Since 2002, funding for health care has continued to be collected centrally but is then allocated, following some minor adjustments, on a per capita basis to the 17 regions. The regional governments can use their own revenues to allocate additional funds to health. They are responsible for ensuring that there is universal health care coverage and that there is adequate provision of health care by public or private institutions. Health care workers working in public hospitals and primary care centres are employed by the regional health services.

These changes have had major implications for the Ministry of Health and, since 2002, its role has been limited to initiating national health legislation, defining a basic package of health services, coordinating the activities of the regions, and certain technical activities such as regulating pharmaceuticals. The national government is also responsible for the regulation of education, training and labour conditions and determines the number of places for medical and nursing education. However, certain responsibilities of the Ministry of Education have also been transferred to the regions, which have now become responsible for curriculum design and for financing and supervision of public universities.

The legal basis for coordination of regional health services, seeking to ensure equal access to health services following decentralization, is the Law on the Cohesion and Quality of the Spanish Health Service, enacted in May 2003. The law established the National Commission on Human Resources, charged with providing guidance on the training of health care professionals, continuing professional development, evidence-based care, and quality assurance.

Workforce supply

Mechanisms for planning human resources in Spain over recent decades have suffered from many weaknesses, resulting in serious imbalances between the educational sector and the labour market.

There is no comprehensive information system to monitor the actual number of health care workers in Spain. The professional associations, for example, hold information on how many members they have, but since 2000, membership has ceased to be obligatory. In addition, those who have retired are not being removed from the registers. There is thus some contention about whether there are too many or too few doctors in Spain (Cooper 1996; O'Neil 1997; Bosch 1999; Peters 1999). While the emergence of unemployment since the 1980s in the medical profession points to an oversupply of physicians, Spain remains below the European average in terms of employment in the health sector. According to data supplied to the OECD, employment in the health sector as a percentage of total employment in Spain in 2002 was the lowest ratio of all OECD countries; at 4.3%, it compared with an average of 6.9% in the European Economic Area (OECD 2003).

While the number of dentists in Spain was far below the European average in 1985, it has since increased by more than 200%. According to the registers of professional associations, there were 0.4 physicians, 0.5 nurses and 0.04 pharmacists per 1000 population in 2000. There has been an increasing participation of women in the medical profession (See Table 9.1).

As shown in Table 9.1, the number of nurses in Spain has remained far below the European average, with a resulting ratio of nurses to doctors much lower

Table 9.1 *Members of professional associations in Spain, 1985–2000*

	1985			2000		
	Absolute number	Rate per 100 000 population	Women	Absolute number	Rate per 100 000 population	Women
Physicians	127 195	331 (313)	25.3%	179 033	435 (355)	37.8%
Pharmacists	29 969	78 (52)	56.9%	50 759	123 (50)	66.8%
Dentists	5 137	13 (39)	14.2%	17 538	43 (50)	37.0%
Nurses	143 508	380 (707)	72.8%	204 485	497 (705)	80.5%

Sources: Professional associations, National Institute of Statistics and European Health for All database.
Note: The European average is given in parentheses.

than in other European countries. In 2000, this ratio was 1.14, almost half the European average of 1.99.

According to the Labour Force Survey undertaken by the National Institute of Statistics, 130 000 doctors and 147 000 nurses were employed in the Spanish health system in 2002, the great majority in the public sector. The number of health care workers in Spain has increased significantly in the last two decades. Between 1991 and 2001, the number of physicians who were members of medical associations increased by 20.4%, far surpassing the growth of the Spanish population in the same period (5.1%). There are significant geographical variations. The region of Aragon has 0.6 doctors per 1000 population, while the region of Ceuta y Melilla (two Spanish enclaves on the coast of North Africa) has only 0.3.

Accurate data on the number of specialists are lacking. The Ministry of Health and the Ministry of Education register degrees awarded in the health sciences, which serves as official accreditation for practice, but they do not remove inactive or deceased physicians from their registers. Furthermore, in response to growing unemployment among specialists, many doctors have pursued several specializations. The specialization rate in Spain is very high, as all physicians in the hospital sector now have to specialize to gain employment. There are more than two specialists for every general practitioner. In most specialties, the number of specialists exceeds current needs. However, the age distribution of specialists is extremely uneven, with a study undertaken in 1997 finding that 11 specialties had more than half of their members between 42 and 51 years of age (Gonzalez 1997).

The geographical distribution of specialists is very uneven across the country's regions. Excluding the specialty of family medicine, in 1997 there were only 114 specialists per million population in the region of Extremadura, compared with 219 specialists in Madrid. Territorial inequalities were most pronounced for dentists. In those 10 regions that were under the responsibility of INSALUD in 2001, the region with the highest level of provision had 3.7 more dentists than the region with the lowest ratio of dentists to population. There are also regional inequalities in the provision of family doctors, which have increased over the last decade. The number of children served by each paediatrician ranged from 824 in Asturias to 1603 in Castilla-La Mancha. In addition to disparities at regional level, there are more doctors in major cities where teaching hospitals are located than in rural areas (Gonzalez 2001). However, reflecting the extent of unemployment among doctors, even in rural municipalities doctors' positions are generally filled.

One of the main driving forces behind the supply of specialist doctors is the need of hospitals for the cheap labour provided by physicians training to become specialists. Positions for specialization are opened by hospitals to meet this demand and to gain status as a teaching hospital, rather than to meet the future need for specialists.

At the end of the 1990s, about 65% of health care workers were employed in hospitals. The share of female doctors has increased in recent years. In 2000, 66.3% of medical students were female, compared with 37.8% of members of the professional association for physicians. In 2003, only 35% of university professors in health sciences were women.

A reform of primary health care was initiated in 1984. Having previously worked mainly in single practices, most general practitioners now work in interdisciplinary teams in publicly owned primary care centres. In 2002, 0.7 physicians per 1000 population were working in the public primary care sector, compared to 1.2 physicians working in public hospitals. Primary care and family medicine continue to be less valued among physicians than hospital medicine, reflecting differences in salary levels and the hospital-centred system of training of physicians. Furthermore, there was a relative decline in employment in primary care between 1992 and 2000. In 2000, each primary care doctor attended to 21.1% more patients than in 1992. Doctors are reacting to these increasing pressures by referring patients more rapidly to specialized care, with the consequence that primary care is undermined even further.

Traditionally, migration of Spanish doctors has been limited. In the 1980s and early 1990s, some specialists were recruited to Spain. Since then, the migratory flow has changed and Spanish specialists are now emigrating to nearby countries such as Portugal. In 2000, an agreement facilitating employment was signed between Spain and the United Kingdom. In the United Kingdom, salaries are more than double those in Spain, but the exact extent of migration from Spain is unknown.

In 2000, there were 204 485 members of nursing associations, equivalent to 0.5 per 1000 population, although this figure includes physiotherapists and midwives. According to the Labour Force Survey, 72.1% were working. The geographical distribution is more uneven than that of physicians who are members of medical associations. There is a more than twice the difference between the regions with the lowest and highest ratios of nurses to population. In Murcia, there were 0.37 nurses per 1000 population, compared to 0.79 in Navarra. Nurse specialization has had limited development in Spain. In 2000, only 6.5% of nurses who were members of professional associations had a specialty, with midwifery, pursued by 3.1% of all nurses, being the most common. As the rate of unemployment among nurses is not very high, there has been little emigration of nurses.

Health care management is not yet a profession in Spain, so that health managers are generally drawn from other professions, such as medicine, law or economics. Often, the appointment of managers rewards political loyalty rather than professional competence. Spanish hospitals typically have two senior management positions: the medical director and the hospital manager. The medical director facilitates the communication between medical staff and the hospital manager and is responsible for the management of clinical processes. Management positions at an intermediate level are generally filled by non-clinically trained managers, responsible for accounting and budget management. The proportion of health managers who are physicians has increased in recent decades. Currently, about 40% of managers in hospitals and 50% in primary care centres are physicians, most of whom are male.

The number of health care managers has increased spectacularly in the last two decades, partly as a result of political decentralization, as each region has created its own health care administration. Overall, health managers constitute 1.5% of hospital personnel. In general, there is a persisting lack of under-standing between managers and medical staff.

Education and training

The Ministry of Health, in conjunction with the Ministry of Education, regulates the undergraduate and postgraduate training of medical professionals. Most health care professionals are trained in public universities and training centres. Fees for registration and credits in public universities are moderate and total fees for one year of medical studies are about €1000. About 27.5% of students receive scholarships, which in 2001 amounted on average to €613 per year. There has, however, been an increasing contribution from private universities in recent years, often offering courses involving a shorter duration of study.

University degree programmes in Spain either follow a short course of three years or a long course of four and more years. In 2003/2004, 19% of students on shorter courses and 11% of students on longer courses studied in private universities.

The medical and pharmacy curricula are quite similar in all universities in Spain. A degree in medicine or pharmacy requires six years of study. The first three years are pre-clinical and classroom-based, while in most of the final year teaching takes place in accredited training hospitals.

The number of university places is determined by the National University Commission, which is accountable to the Ministry of Education and includes representatives of all universities. To enter university, students have to complete compulsory education until the age of 16, complete two additional school years and then achieve a certain score in the university entrance examinations (known as PAU). It is also possible to gain access to university through vocational training, but the required scores are considerably higher. Entry is based on results from both school and university entrance examinations. Degrees in health sciences are in high demand and dropout rates are low. In general, there are more than three applications for each university place on offer but this figure increases to 5.15 for medicine and 5.7 for physiotherapy.

The country's medical schools have dramatically reduced their number of places since 1979. At that time, there were no entry restrictions and 20 000–24 000 students enrolled in undergraduate medical studies each year. This number has now been reduced to about 4000 per year.

The medical undergraduate curriculum is focused on diseases seen in hospital. Of a total of 562 credits, only 15 compulsory credits are devoted to public health, epidemiology, primary care and health education. Training in pharmacology is only vaguely related to the actual practice of writing prescriptions (Baos Vincente 1999). There is a need to respond to the changing professional roles and responsibilities of doctors, with greater emphasis on ethics, research methods, and interdisciplinary teamwork (Segovia de Arana, Pera et al. 1999).

Since 1995, in compliance with European Union regulations enacted in 1991, all physicians in Spain must undertake a specialization after their medical studies in order to work in the public sector. As a result, almost every medical graduate, including those aiming to work in general practice, undertakes a specialization. The Ministry of Health, the regional governments and the National Council for Specialists, representing the professions, reach a joint decision on the number of annual openings for specialists.

As a result of the introduction of compulsory specialization, the universities have lost their right to accredit doctors. They enter agreements with teaching hospitals with regard to the clinical training of medical students and student nurses, but do not play a role in specialist training. Universities have also lost their leadership in health research. Biomedical research is now mainly carried out in hospitals, which have established increasingly well-funded research units.

The curriculum for the specialization of doctors has become increasingly centralized over the last two decades. Programmes and content of specialization are standardized across the country and there is a single national entrance examination. Since 1988, private centres have been accredited to act as teaching facilities. Each year, openings for specialization are announced for all 48 medical specialties. In accredited training hospitals, specializing students provide the backbone of the duty shifts, offering hospitals a cheap workforce, as already mentioned. The hospitals therefore have no incentive to limit the openings of specialist positions. Currently, there are more positions for specialization than graduate medical students.

National commissions decide the training programmes for each specialization, the training period and the number of vacancies offered each year. The commissions comprise representatives of scientific societies, university lecturers, health professionals, residents and medical colleges. For the academic year 2003/ 2004, 5518 positions for specialization were announced, 68% of which were for specialties other than family medicine. In 1998, Spain had 13 590 doctors training as specialists. Specialization lasts three to six years, with the longest period of training for surgery.

In the early 1980s, the specialty of family medicine was created. In this specialization, physicians undertake a three-year residency divided between a hospital and an accredited primary care centre. This innovation has raised the professional status of doctors in primary care. Since 1995, medical students aiming to work in the public primary care sector are required to specialize in family and community medicine. Places for specialization are allocated according to university exam grades and, reflecting its low status, family medicine has the lowest requirements, so that many students with low grades have little option but to specialize in family medicine. In addition, the professional profiles among health care workers in primary care are not well defined (Molina Duran 1996; Gallo Vallejo 1999).

Until 1995, in order to become a dentist, students had to complete a degree in medicine and then specialize during three years of additional studies in stomatology. Since 1995, a specific university degree has been established to comply with EU directives and the number of students and graduates has increased. Dental care is generally not covered by the Spanish national health system, although since 1990 some regions have started programmes of dental health provision for children.

A considerable number of physicians work in public health departments at central, regional or municipal level. While public health is a specialty requiring a residence training programme, in 2002, doctors with at least five years of specialized work were allowed to obtain the public health specialization through an exam. In the last two decades, public health schools have opened in several regions, but they are still lacking national accreditation.

The participation rate of doctors in continuing medical education is very high (Pardell, Ramos et al. 1995; Saturno 1999). Until the late 1990s, training was offered by an array of public and private organizations. In 1998, a national commission was created to certify continuing training in the health sector, while in 2003 an accreditation organization was created.

No other university degree can rival medicine for the number of postgraduate and doctoral students. In 2000/2001, there were 9500 students carrying out their doctoral studies in medicine, constituting 15% of all doctoral students. 26.1% of doctoral students in medicine were women.

Courses for health managers have been offered for several decades at the National School of Health (*Escuela Nacional de Sanidad*). Physiotherapy, previously a specialty within nursing, became an independent degree in 1983/1984, followed by odontology in 1986, optometry in 1988, occupational therapy in 1991 and speech therapy in 1992.

Nursing and physiotherapy are short-course programmes. Prior to the 1970s, nurses followed a technical two-year course, placed at hospitals without university links. Since the late 1970s, nursing was upgraded to a degree course. Whether or not the teaching of nursing should be upgraded into a long-term course is currently being considered; this would mean that nurses could continue into postgraduate studies. Alicante University has introduced this more advanced course, but it is not yet nationally recognized. The only post-graduate programmes for nurses currently recognized are mental health and midwifery, both introduced in 1996.

The training of auxiliary nurses, assistants and laboratory technicians takes place in vocational training schemes outside the university. Training programmes at technical training centres last two years and do not require the certificate for admission to university, but can be started after completing secondary school at the age of 16. The programmes are funded by the Ministry of Education.

Working conditions

Many physicians and nurses have labour rights similar to civil servants, including the "ownership" of their position, a regulation dating back to the Franco era. There are currently 135 000 health care workers in the public sector with "statutory" status (*personal estatutario*). Applicants have to pass an examination to gain access to public employment, but once they have passed this exam, they are in effect granted a permanent position. However, one of the main obstacles for health care workers in the last decade was the lack of stable employment. In 2000, approximately 40% of medical personnel were interns. Following several strikes, new civil service posts were opened in 2002 and 2003. A few months before the transfer of health care responsibilities to the 10 regions where it had previously been under the umbrella of INSALUD, about 37 000 positions were opened for health care professionals in these regions.

There have been a number of conflicting regulations concerning public health care workers. The Law for Health Professions, passed in December 2003, was the first general regulation on human resources in the health sector to be established in recent decades. The law regulated the career path of physicians and nurses and introduced some significant changes in salary matters. However, it was considered to be vague and has failed to change the status quo significantly.

Primary care centres include multidisciplinary teams comprising general physicians, paediatricians, nurses, a social worker and administrative support staff. The primary care team provides an integrated package of care, covering primary and preventive care, health promotion and rehabilitation services. Each team is led by a physician who assumes medical responsibility for the services provided.

Public hospitals are organized into departments or units comprising medical teams. Some hospital departments are further divided into sections. Specialist care outside hospitals is provided in clinics, where specialists work on an individual basis. Many doctors in public hospitals also work in the private sector. The working day in hospitals generally lasts from 8 am to 3 pm from Monday to Friday, leaving scope for private practice. Efforts to keep doctors in the public sector on a full-time basis have not been successful. The Law for Health Professions of 2003 transposed the EU Working Time Directive into domestic legislation, establishing a maximum working time of 48 hours per week. Currently, however, this directive is not fully applied in the health sector in any region of Spain.

Salaries in the national health system vary according to region. A fixed salary is determined by the central government, while a variable pay scheme is determined by the regional health services. In all regions except Catalonia, doctors can earn a supplementary allowance if they agree to work exclusively in the public sector, amounting on average to 25% of the fixed salary. In 2001, the salary of a specialist working non-exclusively in the public health sector with 12 years' experience and four 24-hour duties was about €44 179. The Law for Health Professions of 2003 introduced a new supplementary allowance based on the professional level achieved. There is a considerable disparity in gross earnings across regions. In 2002, a hospital specialist in Catalonia received €45 037, while the salary in Navarra was €52 990. Physicians in specialist training in the INSALUD regions in 2001 earned €11 678 in the first year and €16 041 in the fifth year. The decentralization of health care organization has resulted in salary increases for all specialties.

The salary of specialists working in primary care is in some regions up to 15% dependent on capitation, i.e. patient numbers and age. In some regions, additional allowances are allocated for working in remote rural areas. The total earnings of a primary care specialist with 12 years' experience and four monthly duties were approximately €41 000 in 2001, remaining below the salaries of specialists working in hospitals.

Job satisfaction levels among doctors are low. A survey carried out in Madrid in 2003 with 1554 participating physicians found that more than half would change their profession, given the opportunity. One-third claimed to have suffered some form of harassment and many women reported having faced discrimination. There are a number of reasons for the lack of motivation among health care workers, including inadequate opportunities for professional development.

As with doctors, nurses have permanent employment status in the public health sector. Nursing has become increasingly autonomous and better defined in the last two decades, but the professional functions of nurses are not well distinguished from those of doctors or auxiliary staff. The professional associations of nurses frequently complain that nurses are merely treated as assistants to physicians.

The salaries of nurses differ between regional health authorities, as each negotiates the variable part of salaries and other working conditions, such as the working time per week, with the respective trade unions. Nurses can increase their salaries by working in shifts. In the regions covered by INSALUD in 2001, nurses in secondary and tertiary care received a fixed salary of €17 517 per year, while nurses in primary care received a fixed salary of €19 019 per year.

Performance management

Managers have little autonomy in the management of human resources, owing to the inflexibility of employment regulations. The relevant legislation is rigid, ignores regional differences and acts as a barrier to the implementation of modern human resources policies. That many physicians work in both the public and the private sector further decreases the efficiency of the system. Productivity of doctors and nurses is particularly low, as there are no appropriate incentives for improving performance. The individual economic incentives offered so far have created conflicts between colleagues, a bad working atmosphere and suspicions of arbitrariness. Necessary reforms are being blocked by trade unions and professional associations.

In recent years, regional health authorities have entered into annual contracts with public hospitals and health centres that contain objectives in terms of cost-efficiency and the quality of care. These contracts have now become the norm for the majority of public hospitals and primary care centres. They have helped to decentralize budget management, increase the participation of professionals and improve information systems (Meneu 2000). Many new hospitals were set up as public sector companies rather than as public bodies. They offer their employees conventional labour agreements, which allows for more flexibility in the management of human resources.

There has also been an attempt to professionalize the management of health services and to increase the autonomy of health managers. Since the mid-1990s, new systems for the recruitment of health managers have been introduced, contracting out the politically charged selection process. However, there is much left to do in terms of the modernization of management.

Nearly all regions of Spain have officially embraced the goal of improving the quality of health services. The Law on the Cohesion and Quality of the Spanish Health Service of 2003 created the Quality Assurance Agency, charged with the development of standards and the accreditation of hospitals as referral centres of the national health service. As already mentioned, the Ministry of Health accredits hospitals that offer specialist training. It is also involved in the accreditation of hospitals for teaching at undergraduate level. In recent years, an increasing number of hospitals and primary care centres have sought voluntary accreditation by independent agencies.

Regulation

Regulation of human resources in health is vested in different levels of the public administration. As already mentioned, the central state has the main responsibility for undergraduate and postgraduate training and sets out the policies for civil servants. The central government also establishes the national budget for health, which is then distributed among the regions.

Many responsibilities for human resources in Spain, however, now belong to the regional governments, which have become responsible for defining the optional content of curricula and for financing and evaluating their universities. They can also allocate additional funds for health. The Interterritorial Council for the National Health System, including representatives from the central and regional governments, is charged with securing a consensus between central and regional political actors.

Conclusions

So far, human resources planning in Spain has taken a short-term perspective, resulting in serious imbalances between the supply of and the demand for health care workers. There are currently too many specialists and the ratio of nurses to doctors is very low compared to the European average. It will also be necessary to put more emphasis on primary care, to better define the professional role of nurses, and to modernize management structures. The status of health care workers as civil servants has acted as another brake on the development of modern human resources policies.

Overall, there are too many institutions with different interests involved in the process of decision-making on human resources in the health sector. In the present situation, it is difficult to gain consensus on the necessary number of physicians or nurses and to coordinate the centralized regulation of education, training and working conditions with the decentralized provision of health care.

REFERENCES

Baos Vincente V (1999). La calidad en la prescripción de medicamentos [Quality in medical prescribing]. *Información Terapeutica del Sistema Nacional de Salud,* 23(2): 45–54.

Bosch X (1999). Too many physicians trained in Spain. *JAMA,* 282(11): 1025–1026.

Cooper RA (1996). Unemployed physicians. *New England Journal of Medicine* 334(8): 541–542.

Gallo Vallejo FJ (1999). El perfil profesional del médico de familia. El grupo de trabajo de la Sociedad Española de Medicina Familiar y Comunitaria [The professional profile of the family doctor. Working group of the Spanish Society of Family and Community Medicine]. *Atención Primaria,* 23(4): 236–248.

Gonzalez B (1997). El mercado laboral sanitario y sus consecuencias en la formacion. Numerus clausus [The labour market and its consequences for professional medical training]. In: *La formacion de los profesionales de la salud [Medical education].* Bilbao, Edita Fundacion BBV: 428–467.

Gonzalez B (2001). *Evaluación de las políticas de servicios sanitario en el estado de las autonomias. Organización y gestión [Evaluation of health care policies within independent regions. Organization and management]. Vol. II, part 3*. Barcelona, G. Lopez i Casasnovas, Fundación BBV: 15–233.

Meneu R (2000). Formación de dirección por objetivos y Contratos–Programa [Management training and development by means of target and the Contracts Programme]. *Revista Valenciana de Medicina de Familia*, 6.

Molina Duran F (1996). Perfil profesional del personal de atención primaria. Un studio Delphi [Professional profile of primary care personnel]. *Atención Primaria*, 17(1): 24–32.

OECD (2003). *Health data 2003*. Paris, Organisation for Economic Co-operation and Development (http://www.oecd.org).

O'Neil EH (1997). Are there too many physicians? *Hospital Practice*, 32(9): 146–148.

Pardell H et al. (1995). Los medicos y la formación medica continuada. Resultados de una encuesta realizada in Cataluna [Doctors and continuing medical education. Results of a survey conducted in Catalonia]. *Anales de Medicina Interna*, 12(4): 168–174.

Peters B (1999). Physician supply and demand in the new millennium. *Michigan Health and Hospitals*, 35(3): 18–19.

Rico A (2000). *Health care systems in transition: Spain*. Copenhagen, WHO Regional Office for Europe, on behalf of the European Observatory on Health Care Systems.

Saturno PJ (1999). Training for quality management: a report on a nationwide distance learning initiative for physicians in Spain. *International Journal of Quality in Health Care*, 11(1): 67–71.

Segovia de Arana J et al. (1999). *La formación de los profesionales de la salud [Medical education]*. Informe Fundacion BBV.

Chapter 10

United Kingdom

James Buchan, Alan Maynard

Setting the context

In the United Kingdom, most health care is organized and delivered through the National Health Service (NHS). The NHS is funded from general taxation and is free at the point of delivery. More than one million staff, most of them organized in trade unions, are working in several hundred hospitals and primary care units. Private-sector provision of health care is mainly confined to care and nursing homes and a small but expanding acute sector, both of which are largely funded from public sources.

This chapter focuses on England, the largest of the countries constituting the United Kingdom. Since political devolution in 1998, the other three countries of the United Kingdom, Northern Ireland, Wales and Scotland, have assumed legislative responsibility for health policy. While there are some variations, all NHS health professionals are registered at the United Kingdom level, and most aspects of human resources policy, in particular contract and remuneration conditions, are similar.

Reforming the NHS

Over the last 15 years there have been two attempts to reform the NHS; the first by the Conservative Governments of 1991–1997, the second by the Labour Government, in power since May 1997. Human resources were dealt with very differently in the two reform packages. The Thatcher reforms of the 1990s pursued the decentralization of managerial responsibility and the creation of an internal market. However, workforce planning and human resources were not explicitly considered within the programme of reforms and the pace of change was slow.

The election of the Labour Government in May 1997 led to a further reorganization of the NHS. Human resources are now explicitly highlighted as a key element for improving the quantity and quality of health service delivery. In addition to radical changes in the contracts for general practitioners and hospital consultants, a total restructuring of the pay system for other NHS staff is being implemented (DoH 2003).

The NHS Plan

In 2002, total health expenditure in the United Kingdom was 7.7% of GDP, compared to 9.1% in the countries constituting the European Union before May 2004 and 6.5% in Europe as a whole (WHO 2005). In 2000, the Government of the United Kingdom made a commitment to raise expenditure to "the European average", with a projected increase of 7.5% in real terms in each of the next five years after 2002 (DoH 2002).

The focus of health sector reform has been the NHS Plan, which sets out a series of national targets and priorities. The NHS Plan in England was launched in 2000 and covered an initial period of five years, subsequently extended to 2008. The emphasis is on establishing and achieving health gain targets and reinforcing a performance-based management culture. This approach recognizes the need to involve health care staff in decision-making and to ensure that they are appropriately skilled and deployed in sufficient numbers.

Human resources issues

Shortages of skilled staff have been highlighted as one of the main obstacles to achieving NHS targets. A report issued in 2002 stressed that "the UK does not have enough doctors and nurses" (Wanless 2002). The response by the Government has been an explicit commitment to increase the NHS workforce. The human resources element of the NHS Plan is set out in the national NHS human resources strategy "HR in the NHS: more staff, working differently" (DoH 2002).

Reorganization of the NHS workforce planning system in England began in 2002. Locally, Workforce Development Confederations are the key bodies for workforce planning in the NHS in England. They bring together NHS and non-NHS employers to plan and develop the health sector workforce and to make decisions on allocation of funding for training and education.

Box 10.1 *NHS Plan Targets (England)*

NHS Plan targets for staff increase by 2004:

- 7500 more consultants and 2000 more GPs.
- 20 000 more nurses and over 6500 more therapists.
- 5500 more nurses and midwives trained each year.
- 4450 more therapists and other key professional staff trained.
- 1000 more medical school places by 2005 (in addition to the 1100 already announced).
- 550 more GP registrars and 1000 more specialist registrars.

Source: DoH 2002.

At national level, the National Workforce Development Board provides oversight of the workforce strategy required to deliver the NHS Plan. It takes advice from experts on the Workforce Numbers Advisory Board and from seven Care Group Workforce Teams. The latter take a national view of the workforce issues in their care areas, looking across staff groups and sectors. They are responsible for identifying effective ways of training, educating and deploying staff to deliver improvements in services. In this way the Department of Health (DoH) is looking at the long-term future of the health care workforce (DoH 2002).

Workforce supply

As noted above, the main driver for NHS reform has been the NHS Plan of 2000 which included a commitment to increase NHS staffing. This has been set out in a series of specific targets (see Box 10.1).

The targets were not, however, based on any detailed evidence base or the outcome of a planning exercise; they were primarily a political pledge and a means of focusing policy attention. In addition, the targets were presented in terms of headcount rather than whole time equivalent, which may not give an accurate picture of the actual change in available staffing.

In terms of the number of health care workers, recent years have seen a growth in the main NHS staff groups. There has been considerable success in meeting the target for nurses, and policy attention is now focused on allied health professionals (AHPs) and medical staff, as it appears that the Department of Health will face a greater challenge in meeting the targets for these groups (Table 10.1).

Health care assistants are a relatively new addition to the NHS workforce. They are vocationally qualified workers who provide support to health professionals; many are supervised by nurses. The traditional support worker

Table 10.1 *Number of NHS staff by selected occupation, NHS England, 1999 and 2002 (headcount)*

	1999	**2002**
Medical and dental staff	70 000	77 031
Health care assistants	22 576	32 873
Unqualified nursing	116 791	123 672
Qualified nursing	310 142	346 537
Qualified allied health professionals	47 920	53 455
Managers	24 287	32 294

Source: DoH Statistical Bulletin 2003/2, June 2003.

for qualified nurses were nursing auxiliaries, termed "unqualified nursing" in DoH data.

Doctors

The NHS stock of physicians is growing from a low level, when compared to the European average. In the United Kingdom there were only 2.1 physicians per 1000 population in 2002, compared to a European average of 3.5 per 1000 population (WHO 2005). In the English NHS, there were 71 251 physicians in 2002, an increase from 50 381 in 1992. The gender balance is changing, with increasing numbers of women entering medicine; the percentage of female general practitioners increased to nearly 35% in 2002. Increasingly, other skill groups are used in the delivery of primary care, including nurses as well as receptionists and managers.

Tables 10.2. and 10.3. show the distribution of hospital specialists and general practitioners across the countries of the United Kingdom. The ratio of physicians to population is lower in England than in the rest of the United Kingdom as a result of differential funding of the United Kingdom's constituent countries.

Nurses and midwives

There are approximately 640 000 nurses and midwives on the United Kingdom professional register. Of these, about 400 000 are employed in the NHS, and about 100 000 in other jobs and sectors, with the remainder not currently employed in nursing (Buchan and Seccombe 2003). OECD data on the ratio of nurses to population suggest that the United Kingdom has fewer nurses than many other developed countries. However, these data may overestimate the number of nurses in other countries as, unlike the situation in the United Kingdom, whose data refer to NHS full-time equivalents, data from other countries are often headcounts, and may include nurses working in other sectors or all nurses on the register.

Table 10.2 *Number of general practitioners per 1000 population*

	1992	1997	2002
England	0.59	0.61	0.63
Wales	0.61	0.65	0.66
Scotland	0.75	0.78	0.84
Northern Ireland	0.63	0.62	0.63

Source: Office of Health Economics, Compendium of Health Statistics, 2003.

Table 10.3 *Number of medical and dental staff in hospitals per 1000 population*

	1992	1997	2001
England	0.91	1.12	1.25
Wales	0.95	1.15	1.28
Scotland	1.21	1.44	1.55
Northern Ireland	1.37	1.29	1.35

Source: Office of Health Economics, Compendium of Health Statistics, 2003.

Table 10.4 *Whole time equivalent in the NHS Qualified Nursing and Midwifery Workforce, 1999–2002*

	1999	2002
England	250 651	279 287
Scotland	35 494	37 216
Wales	17 397	18 766
Northern Ireland	11 207	11 933

Sources: DoH Statistical Bulletin 2003/2; Northern Ireland – DHSSPSNI 2002 workforce census; Scotland data – ISD Workforce Statistics 2003; Wales – Wales Health Statistics and Analysis Unit.
Note: % figures are rounded.

In the area of nursing it is apparent that meeting the staffing target in the NHS Plan may be a measure of political commitment, but it is not based on a comprehensive system of human resource planning and does not guarantee the effective deployment of the nursing workforce. National targets need to be underpinned by workforce planning, taking account of changing service plans, health needs and funding (Buchan and Seccombe 2003; Welsh Assembly 2003). The most recent comparable workforce data for the United Kingdom show an increase in nurse staffing (see Table 10.4).

Two interventions have been critical in achieving the staffing growth in England: international recruitment and "returners". The DoH in England has supported the international recruitment of nurses as a method of achieving staffing growth. There has been a steep growth in the level of international recruitment of nurses in recent years, as shown in Figure 10.1. In 2001–02, there were 15 064 new entrants to the United Kingdom register from non-EU

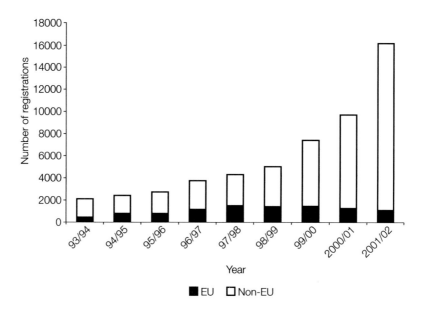

Figure 10.1 *Admissions to the UKCC Register from EU Directive/non-EU sources: 1993/1994–2001/2002 (initial registrations)*

countries and 1091 from the EU. For the first time, there were more new entrants from non-United Kingdom sources than there were new graduates from the United Kingdom.

The main non-EU sources in 2001/02 were the Philippines (7235), South Africa (2114) and Australia (1342). Immigration from India and Zimbabwe has also significantly increased. International recruitment was initially portrayed as a short-term stopgap but has become an integral part of recruitment to the NHS in England.

Encouraging nurses to return to NHS employment has been another key element of NHS policy. In April 2001, a "returner package" was introduced in England, providing free refresher training and financial support. Similar initiatives were undertaken in the other United Kingdom countries. Data on returners to England suggest that on average about 3700 nurses, midwives and health visitors have annually returned to work in recent years.

Although overall nursing numbers have increased, it is less clear whether the growing number of nurses are in the "right" place or have the "right" skills. Headline growth masks significant variations within different NHS nursing specialties and grades. The increase in NHS nursing headcount figures for England between 1999 and 2002 has mainly been among general nurses and nurse managers, while there has been a decrease in the number of district nurses and health visitors (see Table 10.5).

Table 10.5 *Number of qualified nurses and midwives, NHS England, 1999 and 2002 (headcount)*

	1999	2002
Nurse consultant	–	330
Manager	4 821	5 784
Paediatric nurse	10 826	12 288
Regular midwife	22 799	23 249
Health visitor	12 800	12 774
District nurse	14 258	13 393
First level regular nurse	218 817	255 712
Second level regular nurse	25 821	18 450
Total qualified	310 142	346 537

Source: DoH Statistical Bulletin 2003/2, June 2003.

Allied health professionals

Allied health professionals form a category of NHS employees that includes a range of therapeutic and scientific staff groups. In contrast to nursing, where there had been significant reductions in the numbers entering training in the 1990s and little growth in the NHS workforce, the AHP workforce was already growing in numbers prior to the NHS Plan. For therapists and other key health professionals, the numbers entering training had increased from 4690 in 1996/7 to 6600 in 2000/01. For all AHP groups, there was a target of recruiting 6500 more therapists and other health professionals by 2004, although with no specific growth rates envisaged for any one occupation.

Within the AHP group, all occupations have reported significant staffing growth since 1995, with the exception of chiropody. The other scientific, therapeutic and technical occupations have also reported staffing growth, with the exception of pathology. The increase in the workforce is driven by new, mainly young recruits, resulting in a relatively young age profile in these occupations.

Summary

While some of the short-term staffing targets in the NHS Plan have already been met, questions remain. Staff shortages are not uniformly distributed throughout the NHS. The NHS in the south-east of England, particularly London, continues to experience staffing difficulties (Buchan et al. 2003). The United Kingdom is improving its workforce planning infrastructure, but continues to lack adequate information about imbalances between supply and demand and the causes and possible remedies for these deficiencies. How can we be sure that 20 000 or 35 000 more nurses will be sufficient when a comprehensive needs assessment is lacking? Will there be too many doctors in 2012 when medical schools produce more physicians and nurses have taken over medical tasks (Walker and Maynard 2003)?

Education and training

Pre-registration training of health professionals in the United Kingdom is funded by the Government and delivered by public sector education institutions and universities. The United Kingdom Government therefore has a number of policy levers to influence the number of trained health professionals.

Programmes for those in training or professional education are currently being altered in an attempt to broaden the recruitment base. Key features include more flexible curricula and extended accreditation of prior learning. New avenues into medical education are being developed, while the number of places in medical schools is being increased. There is also an increased interest in interprofessional education. In 2001, the DoH set out its plans for "lifelong learning" for NHS staff, establishing a "Skills Escalator" and an NHS University, although the latter has since been replaced by a new body, the NHS Institute for Innovation and Improvement.

Doctors

A range of policies has been applied to increase the supply of doctors.

1 Entry to medical schools has been increased by 30% by creating new medical schools and increasing entries to existing schools.

2 Changes in skill mix. Nurses are being trained to take over doctors' roles and a new grade of "consultant nurse" is being developed in English hospitals. Outside hospitals, nurses are being trained to dispense pharmaceuticals. While such skill mix changes may compensate for shortages of doctors, they might increase nurse shortages.

3 Incentive systems to enhance recruitment and retention have been put in place.

4 International recruitment. Considerable efforts have been put into recruiting more doctors from overseas. The United Kingdom has traditionally recruited doctors from the Indian subcontinent and the Middle East and over 25% of the existing doctor stock has been trained overseas. The new recruitment drive has focused on countries with a surplus, such as Spain, but despite attempts to avoid recruitment from developing countries, it has also attracted many doctors from countries such as South Africa. A Code of Practice on

international recruitment has now been enacted, although the private sector is not bound by it.

These policies have facilitated an increase in the number of physicians. However, their effectiveness has been reduced by other developments. The EU Working Time Directive and NHS reforms creating a "consultant-led" service have reduced the number of hours worked, making supply deficiencies more evident. In addition, scandals related to medical practice, which have had wide circulation in the national media, appear to have encouraged much greater caution by practitioners, leading to slower processes of care.

Nurses

Following a period of substantial decline over the last decade, in recent years there has been a significant annual increase in the number of newly qualified nurses and midwives entering the United Kingdom register from pre-registration education in the United Kingdom. The number of new entrants from education and training in the United Kingdom decreased from 18 980 in 1990/91 to 12 974 in 1998/99, increasing again to 18 048 in 2002/03.

Working conditions

Sustainable improvements in NHS staff retention and productivity will require improvements in working conditions, job satisfaction, career prospects and pay. A series of initiatives to improve working conditions is being implemented in the United Kingdom. Human resources performance indicators, including staff turnover and absence, are being used as part of the overall performance management system. All NHS organizations in England also have to participate in the "Improving Working Lives" (IWL) accreditation process. IWL sets out a series of related human resources practices, covering flexible and healthy working, access to training, child care provision, and staff involvement (DoH 2001).

The NHS also needs a pay and career structure that is responsive to the needs of individuals and supports the attainment of organizational and individual goals. The current pay system, in some ways unchanged since the NHS was set up in 1948, is viewed by all stakeholders as a blockage to meeting NHS Plan objectives.

Negotiations on a new NHS pay system began in 1999 when the health departments of England, Northern Ireland, Scotland and Wales published the "Agenda for Change". From April 2003, pilot sites in the NHS have been introducing a new pay and job evaluation system. The new system will introduce standardized terms and conditions for all NHS staff. The standard working week will be 37½ hours, with annual leave rising from 27 to 33 days with length of service. There will be pay supplements for all working patterns outside normal hours of work. Staff available "on call" outside their normal working hours will receive a fixed pay supplement. If called into work while on call, they will receive compensation for the work done. New regional allowances will be introduced to replace previous London weighting, fringe allowances and cost of living supplements.

The Royal College of Nursing has estimated that the proposals will result in a basic pay increase for nurses of 15.8% over three years. NHS nurses have previously been paid according to a grading system with nine grades. Most nurses were appointed initially on grade four, with annual increments. Promotion from one grade to the next has normally been achieved through assuming a more senior post. This system has been in operation throughout the NHS.

The payment system for doctors

Since the creation of the NHS, the payment system for doctors has remained largely unchanged with annual increases in remuneration determined by a quasi-autonomous nongovernmental organization, the Pay Review Body. Until 2003, hospital consultants were paid a basic salary together with "distinction awards", a crude form of performance-related pay. They were also allowed to partly contract out from the NHS and earn income from private practice. Since April 2003, most NHS consultants have had a new contract, obliging them to work 40 hours per week for the NHS. This contract was the subject of bitter disputes and has been accepted in part because of steep rises in salary rates: the old starting salary of £54 340 (€78 112) has risen to £65 035 (€93 496), with the top of the scale at £88 000 (€126 511). In addition to their salary, hospital doctors are eligible for a revised distinction award scheme (Maynard and Bloor 2003b).

The new contract for general practitioners, implemented since April 2004, is also costly. It involves the switching of the contract from the individual general practitioner to the practice in which they work. The practice can then pay its general practitioners a salary (nearly 40% have already switched to this basis) or according to the 1948 contract based on capitation payments, fee for service and other elements of remuneration.

A new quality agenda of 10 clinical target areas and rewards for management and holism has become an important element of practice income. They are scored up to a maximum of 1050 points, each of which generates a reward.

For instance, the monitoring and management of hypertension and lipids to achieve specified levels brings explicit financial rewards.

Until recently, general practitioners were obliged to offer complete cover for their patients, 24 hours a day, seven days a week. They now have the option of giving up £6000 (€8622) per annum to be released from this obligation. This new contract is already creating some difficulties with "out of hours" cover, resulting in additional pressure on hospital accident and emergency facilities.

By sharply raising the salaries of consultants and general practitioners, recruitment and retention are likely to be enhanced, with the United Kingdom becoming even more attractive to doctors from abroad. However, the effects of these contracts on activity and outcomes are still unclear. One of the problems with the new general practice contract is that what is not listed in the quality targets may be marginalized.

Performance management

Nursing and other health workers

The United Kingdom is attempting to achieve efficiency gains by introducing new roles and a new skill mix for health workers. This is the most challenging area of current human resources-related interventions, highlighting how a funding increase will not in itself stimulate the type of organizational change that is intended for the NHS.

The "Changing Workforce Programme" (DoH 2001) is the focal point of government-led initiatives to encourage new roles and a new skill mix. It has involved setting up pilot sites where a range of staffing reconfigurations are being evaluated, many underpinned by the introduction of care protocols or pathways.

There are likely to be at least two main areas of attention. The first is to develop the role of nurse practitioner (and other advanced roles for nurses and allied health professionals), to free up physicians. The second is to further develop the role of vocationally qualified health care assistants so as to free up nurses and other health professionals. The Wanless report suggested that nurse practitioners could take on about 20% of work currently undertaken by general practitioners and junior doctors, while health care assistants could cover about 12.5% of nurses' current workload (Wanless 2002).

Doctors

International health care literature casts doubt on the idea that "more means better". Recent American analysis of small area variations in patients presenting with hip fracture, colorectal cancer and acute myocardial infarction, for example, showed that patients in high spending regions had no better survival than those in lower spending regions (Fisher et al. 2003a; Fisher et al. 2003b).

While some of this research has yet to be extended to Europe, variations in clinical practice in the United Kingdom have been well documented. According to data from York University, there was a 60–80% variation in the distribution of local practitioners in general surgery, urology, trauma and orthopaedics, ENT and ophthalmic surgery (Bloor and Maynard 2002).

Although the need for improving performance management at the level of the individual clinician has been recognized, progress has been slow. Data sets are being extended, linking public and private sector and hospitals to death registration data. However, the notion that clinical trust can only survive in a carefully managed framework of performance review is not yet fully accepted (Maynard and Bloor 2003a).

In recent years, increased attention has been devoted to clinical governance, as a framework through which NHS organizations are accountable for continuously improving the quality of their services and safeguarding high standards of care. The concept entails clear lines of accountability, a programme for improvements, policies for managing risk, and the identification and management of poor performance.

Regulation

In the United Kingdom, professional regulation covers education, training, registration and continuing professional development and revalidation. It also includes setting standards for entry into the profession, and determining people's fitness to practice. Each profession is responsible for self-regulation based on a single United Kingdom-wide body, such as the General Medical Council for doctors.

The English Department of Health has noted that "[p]rotecting patients is at the heart of professional regulation" and initiated a programme to change current regulatory arrangements. The changes seek to ensure that "regulatory bodies are more accountable, open and transparent, responsive to change and operate with greater consistency of approach and with better integration between them".

Self-regulation has been a cornerstone of the NHS since its inception, but many commentators argue that there is a need for more effective systems. The Government has remained committed to self-regulation, but is changing the statutory basis of regulation. It set out its objectives in November 1999

(DoH 1999), including clarity of standards, maintaining public confidence, transparency in tackling fitness to practise, and responsiveness to and protection of patients. The NHS Plan sets out the need for regulatory bodies to change so that they:

- are smaller, with greater public and patient representation;

- have "faster, more transparent procedures";

- develop meaningful accountability to the public and the health service.

To support these changes, a Council for the Regulation of Health Care Professionals and a new Health Professions Council have been established. The latter covers the AHPs and will help to extend professional regulation, covering new groups of staff currently not subject to statutory regulation. The National Patient Safety Agency has been established to protect patients and support staff by minimizing the possibilities for clinical error. The Government of the United Kingdom has also published proposals for the reform of the General Medical Council. The General Dental Council will be smaller and have a larger lay membership. All these developments, however, have been slow in relation to stated intentions and the deficiencies of existing workforce planning.

Conclusions

While some of the short-term NHS Plan staffing targets have been met, questions remain about the cost-effectiveness of skill mix changes (e.g. Lankshear et al. 2005) and about regional variations in clinical practice, quality indicators and level of staff shortages. Will meeting the national staffing targets be sufficient? The United Kingdom is improving its workforce planning infrastructure, but remains far short of having adequate information about stocks, flows and effects of incentive structures.

Staff will have to be retained and motivated, and some working practices will have to be changed. This will require an emphasis on partnership between management and staff, in order to improve working lives and to develop a fairer career structure. It will also require considerable investment in measuring and managing clinical practice activities and outcomes.

REFERENCES

Bloor K, Maynard A (2002). Consultants: managing them means measuring them. *Health Service Journal,* December 2002: 10–11.

Buchan J, Finlayson B, Gough P (2003). *In capital health?* London, King's Fund.

Buchan J, Seccombe I (2003). *More nurses, working differently.* London, Royal College of Nursing.

DoH (1999). *Supporting doctors, protecting patients.* London, Department of Health.

DoH (2001). *Working together – learning together.* London, Department of Health.

DoH (2002). *HR in the NHS: more staff, working differently.* London, Department of Health.

DoH (2003). *A modernised NHS pay system.* London, Department of Health.

Fisher E et al. (2003a). The implications of regional variations in Medicare spending. Part 1: The content, quality and accessibility of care. *Annals of Internal Medicine,* 138(4): 273–287.

Fisher E et al. (2003b). The implications of regional variations in Medicare spending. Part 2: Health outcomes and satisfaction with care. *Annals of Internal Medicine, 138(4)*: 288–298.

Lankshear A et al (2005). Nursing challenges: are changes in the nursing role and skill mix improving patient care? *Health Policy Matters,* 10 (http://www.york.ac.uk/healthsciences/pubs/Hpm10.pdf).

Maynard A, Bloor K (2003a). Do those who pay the piper call the tune? *Health Policy Matters,* 8 (http://www.york.ac.uk/healthsciences/pubs/hpm8final.pdf).

Maynard A, Bloor K (2003b). Trust and performance management in the medical marketplace. *Journal of the Royal Society of Medicine,* 96: 532–539.

Walker A, Maynard A (2003). Managing medical workforces: from relative stability to disequilibrium in the UK NHS. *Applied Health Economics and Health Policy,* 2(1): 25–36.

Wanless D (2002). *Securing our future health: taking a long-term view.* London, Public Enquiry Unit, HM Treasury.

Welsh Assembly (2003). *The review of health and social care in Wales.* Cardiff, Welsh Assembly.

WHO (2005). European Health for All database (HFA-DB) [online database]. Copenhagen, WHO Regional Office for Europe.

Index

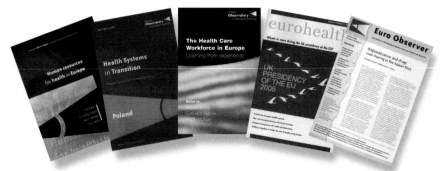

*The European Observatory on Health Systems and Policies
produces a wide range of analytical work on health systems and policies.
Its publishing programme includes:*

☐ **The Health Systems in Transition profiles (HiTs)**. Country-based reports that provide a detailed description of the health systems of European and selected OECD countries outside the region, and of policy initiatives in progress or under development.

HiT profiles are downloadable from: www.euro.who.int/observatory

☐ **Joint Observatory/Open University Press -McGraw Hill Series. A prestigious health series exploring key issues for health systems and policies in Europe.**
Titles include: Mental Health Policy and Practice across Europe ■ Decentralization in Health Care ■ Primary Care in the Driver's Seat ■ Human Resources for Health in Europe ■ Purchasing to Improve Health Systems Performance ■ Social Health Insurance Systems in Western Europe ■ Regulating Pharmaceuticals in Europe

Copies of the books can be ordered from: www.mcgraw-hill.co.uk

☐ **The Occasional Studies**. A selection of concise volumes, presenting evidence-based information on crucial aspects of health, health systems and policies. Recent titles include: Patient Mobility in the EU ■ Private Medical Insurance in the UK ■ The Health Care Workforce in Europe ■ Making Decisions on Public Health ■ Health Systems Transition: learning from experience

Studies are downloadable from: www.euro.who.int/observatory

☐ **Policy briefs**. A series of compact brochures, highlighting key policy lessons on priority issues for Europe's decision-makers, such as cross-border health care, screening, health technology assessment, care outside the hospital.

Policy briefs are downloadable from: www.euro.who.int/observatory

☐ *Eurohealth*. A joint Observatory/LSE Health journal, providing a platform for policy-makers, academics and politicians to express their views on European health policy.

☐ *Euro Observer*. A health policy bulletin, published quarterly, providing information on key health policy issues and health system reforms across Europe.

✶ ✶ ✶ Join our E-Bulletin ✶ ✶ ✶

Are you interested in signing up for the European Observatory's listserve to receive E-Bulletins on news about health systems, electronic versions of our latest publications, upcoming conferences and other news items? If so, please subscribe by sending a blank e-mail to: subscribe-observatory_listserve@list.euro.who.int